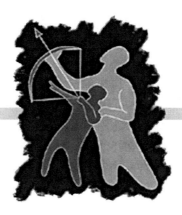

Shoot for the Stars!

A Practical Guide for Helping Your Child Achieve Success in School and the Workplace

Dr. France Morrow

Published by JimSam Inc.
P. O. Box 3363
Riverview, FL 33568
www.JimSamInc.com

1st printing 2008
Printed in the U.S.A.

Shoot for the Stars!

A Practical Guide for Helping Your Child Achieve Success in School and the Workplace represents decades of work designed to help all students who struggle to overcome their *hidden* barriers to academic and vocational success.

I dedicate this book to these students of all ages who have taught me much about the courage, the strength, and the intelligence of students who all too often are written off by educational bureaucracies.

Dr. France Morrow

Important facts for parents, older students, and teachers about *A Practical Guide's* "Basic Program"

The goal of *A Practical Guide* is to raise students' test scores by identifying and removing the "invisible" barriers that nearly half of students struggling with reading and learning need to overcome.

The problem that *A Practical Guide* addresses is that far too many bright students are not able to reach a proficient level in reading, writing, and math. As a result, these students are failing to pass the state standards tests mandated under "No Child Left Behind."

Test proficiency levels are reached when students' barriers to learning are identified and removed. Based on decades of teaching experience and on extensive research into how the brain learns, Dr. France Morrow's Basic Program removes common learning barriers by improving students'

- Working memory
- Attention
- Visual and auditory processing
- Vocabulary

Basic Program results: Parents can expect that with only 24 hours of computer software exercises over six weeks, their children's reading levels can be raised by one, two, three, or more, grade levels. Proficient reading at grade level is recognized by educators as the key to successful learning and to passing the state standards—and other—tests.

Students are surprised to find that the Basic Program is fun and works quickly to raise their ability levels. Here is what *A Practical Guide* students write about their program experiences:

"I love the attention exercises; they are helping to improve my thought process in math."

"I discovered that reading does not have to be a hassle and a stress. With this program I have progressed from a mediocre student into a proficient student. . . . The auditory and visual memory program has helped in my daily classes. . . . The WordSmart program has allowed me access to new vocabulary. I am now able to use more specific language increasing my spoken language as well as written. . . . The Irlen transparencies have altered my view on reading. Before I found myself feeling tired and often sick when I would try to study. With the transparencies I am able to read for hours without a headache or sore eyes."

"[The] brain warm-ups improved my attention and memory capabilities [and] developed a strong foundation for working methods and memorization strategies."

"My eyes do not hurt anymore because I use the overlay provided to me in this program. I find myself reading more and not only to myself, but to my daughter as well. . . . Every time that I started the vocabulary exercises I would learn a new word and many times I would catch myself using that same vocabulary word in class." Note: *This student's reading level improved an amazing 6.5 grade levels from the mid-5th grade level when entering my program to just past the senior year in high school after about 20 hours in the Practical Guide program.*

"[This program brought about] a lot of improvement for memory and attention . . . . I feel more confident in my reading and retaining the information I do read. My comprehension has also improved doing these exercises. . . . In using the applied principles this program has supplied, my class work has improved and my grade point average has increased . . . from a 2.00 to a 3.57."

> *By using A Practical Guide's Basic Program to help very young students, parents and teachers can prevent the development of many reading and learning problems, as well as the stress, anxiety, low self-esteem and behavioral problems that accompany difficulties learning to read. Many students struggle for years into adulthood without knowing what their problems are. Here are two further statements that refer only to the first step in the Basic Program, namely, identification of Irlen Syndrome, or light sensitivity.*

This student was a beginning college student:

"As a child I always wondered what was wrong with me. I had perfect vision and yet the words still appeared blurry. I would start to read a book and would end up falling asleep even when I wasn't tired. I always wondered why. It wasn't until my freshman year in college [this year] that I discovered I had Irlen Syndrome. . . . I would like to take this opportunity to thank Dr. Morrow for allowing me to participate in a program that has enhanced my learning abilities. For once in my life I can say, I enjoy reading."

Finally, here is the remarkable story of a very bright student returning to college for another career path:

"My name is Alice [name changed] and I am 51 years old and pursuing a college business degree. I am enrolled in a psychology class taught by Dr. France Morrow. I mentioned to Dr. Morrow that I was having trouble seeing my accounting homework and psychology labs in the building where I attend classes. I related that the fluorescent lights seemed to bounce off the books I was trying to read and the papers that I was trying to write. Even though I had my vision checked fairly recently and I really did not need reading glasses, I assumed that my vision problems stemmed from the natural changes associated with my age. I tried a number of different strengths of non-prescription glasses and I still experienced the same difficulty seeing white paper under fluorescent lights.

"Dr. Morrow suggested that I might have a problem processing visual cues due to a [genetic] condition called Irlen Syndrome. She gave me the website address for an Irlen Syndrome self-test. She also placed a colored transparency on my psychology test. The fluorescent light stopped bouncing on my psychology test and I was able to concentrate without fighting to read the words through the glare. I immediately experienced a complete reduction in my test anxiety. I also received an A on the test.

"After leaving school that day, I went home and completed the questionnaire on the Irlen Syndrome Website. The list of questions was extensive and surprising in their ability to remind me of the seemingly unrelated difficulties that I have experienced since the day I started kindergarten.

"I am a very motivated and intellectually curious individual. I began trying to read before kindergarten. I could memorize any songs or stories that I heard and repeat them accurately. I loved to read, but not at school. I read at home, in my room with the incandescent light bulb off, and ambient light coming through the curtains of my window. In school, I struggled to be able to put pencil to paper because the words became jumbled up. I lost my place when writing, and then would panic because I could not keep up. I also could not catch a ball or jump rope. Rarely did a week go by that my mother was not called into the school because I had fallen or because I was daydreaming. My teacher showed my mother paper after paper with unacceptable printing or handwriting.

"The Irlen Syndrome test took me on a journey to my past and explained it to me. Sometime this month, I will be going through more testing to find out which transparency colors and tinted lenses will work the best for me.

"[I am writing this] in the hope that it can help make a difference in the lives of others who struggle with the same problems that I have."

Like my student who hopes that her story will help others, I have written A Practical Guide *to help the many students who struggle daily without knowing why they struggle and without knowing that there is help that can open the doors of learning wide for them. If parents and teachers use this Guide's Basic Program to identify and remediate the common reading and learning problems that prevent students from reaching their true potential—and do this at the earliest possible ages, then my hope for this book will be realized.*

France Morrow, Ph.D.

Acknowledgments

I thank my husband Charles for his steadfast belief in me and support of my educational initiatives. The support and collaboration of my friend and colleague Marlene Cousens, a gifted college reading teacher, were critically important during the pilot testing of *A Practical Guide's* Basic Program. I also thank my former colleague Robert Federico, a perceptive therapist and accomplished vocational counselor, now working for Washington State's Department of Social and Health Services. Rob worked with me on implementing my first learning assessment and remediation program; thanks to his skillful direction of the program for our college's Welfare-to-Work students, many adults struggling with reading were able to advance their education and enter the workforce. My colleagues D'Anna Clark and Michelle Orton, certified Irlen screeners, have helped me implement other pilot studies with younger students by identifying the precise colors for the Irlen transparency intervention. Finally, the editing help of my friend and colleague, Dr. Inga Wiehl, an accomplished writer, college professor, and university lecturer was indispensable. As I prepared to bring to fruition in writing the work of many years, Dr. Wiehl helped me clarify the important issues of voice and audience. For her help at a critical juncture, I am most grateful.

I heartily thank all these caring individuals who have joined me in dedicating themselves to the education of struggling students of all ages.

In addition, I am grateful to the Fred Meyer and Allstate Foundations for their generous funding of my pilot study research; earlier programs were funded by the Wal-Mart and Weyerhaeuser Foundations. The Boeing Company contributed to pilot studies with donations of computers and printers.

I thank as well the Washington State University Foundation for administering my grant funding.

Brief Table of Contents

Table of Contents

Preface for parents

Currently flooding the Internet is a veritable tsunami of software exercise programs advertised as improving students' reading and learning abilities. In addition, parents and teachers are besieged with books and programs also advertised as miracle cures for low-performing readers. What, then, can *A Practical Guide* offer that is not now being offered? Although programs and books now being marketed can help some struggling students, there is not a single book or program like the one presented in this *Guide*. What this book uniquely provides parents is a powerful *combination* of assessments and remediations for the most common *invisible barriers* that prevent students from achieving the academic success they deserve.

If parents and their children do not know what is blocking academic success, no amount of extra tutoring, reading, or software exercising can help students reach their full learning potential. Furthermore, the software exercises my Basic Program identifies and recommends for remediating students' hidden barriers are the newest and best evidence-based programs available. My Basic Program builds those cognitive-processing abilities of memory, attention, and vocabulary that are the focus of the most sophisticated computer programs, for example, Scientific Learning's "Fast ForWord," which now is available only to educational institutions and professionals in private practice.

I have spent most of my adult life teaching; my focus is, and always has been, on helping students with learning problems. Over the past two decades I have uncovered the primary invisible, but quite widespread, problems causing very bright and capable students to struggle and often fail to achieve their academic goals. These hidden problems, frequently hidden from students themselves, as well as from their parents and teachers, are first, visual-perceptual and auditory-processing dyslexias; second, problems with memory and attention; and, third, vocabularies inadequate for grade-level reading and learning.

This *Guide* will explain that Irlen Syndrome, essentially a problem involving light sensitivity, is a type of visual-perceptual dyslexia which, when unremediated, can cause students to have working memory and attention problems that make reading such a painful chore that students are prevented from achieving grade-level vocabularies. A growing body of university research evidence is validating the existence of Irlen Syndrome (IS). In Australia, England, and many other European countries, Irlen Syndrome has long been recognized as a critical barrier to student reading achievement.

Across the U.S., many school districts now routinely screen students for IS; many states, among them California, Florida, Massachusetts, Nevada, New Mexico, and Oklahoma permit colored overlays on their standardized tests. The Commonwealth of Massachusetts allows the Irlen intervention of colored overlays when students take the Massachusetts competency exams and teachers take state licensing exams; the State of California has approved the use of colored overlays on all state-wide assessment tests, as has Washington State. The Irlen overlay accommodation can be used in California even if it is not specifically mentioned in a student's individual education plan [IEP]. Acceptance of this effective intervention is growing throughout U.S. school districts and, in fact, throughout the world.

To summarize: My decades of teaching and educational research have led me to the identification of underlying reasons why many students struggle with reading and learning. These often unidentified barriers to learning involve problems with visual and auditory processing, with memory and attention, and with vocabulary. As regards vocabulary, a Gallup survey conducted in 1950 found that the average American fourteen-year-old student's vocabulary contained 25,000 words. When the Gallup Organization replicated this survey in 1999, they found that the average American fourteen-year-old student's vocabulary had shrunk from 25,000 words to a shocking 10,000 words. When students have visual-perceptual and / or auditory dyslexia, they avoid reading and do not develop their vocabularies. This lack of word power makes it difficult for them to pay attention and remember what they hear and see.

In short, *A Practical Guide* is unique in identifying the critical factors—problems with vocabulary, memory, attention, and dyslexia—that prevent students from succeeding.

Furthermore, *A Practical Guide* goes beyond identifying hidden learning barriers and presents effective ways to remediate those critical cognitive-processing problems responsible for the painful academic failure of too many capable, yet struggling, students.

Although cultural factors undoubtedly contribute to the well-publicized failures of American students in the global educational competition, I know that American students do want, and try hard, to succeed academically. However, in classrooms at all levels, I have observed that students, along with their teachers and parents, often do not understand why students are failing to achieve their full potential. *A Practical Guide* provides parents with the means to identify the specific causes for their children's academic problems, as well as providing parents with effective ways to eliminate many hidden barriers with which their children struggle.

Specifically, this *Guide* supplies parents and their children with the free and simple online assessments that will identify Irlen Syndrome, attention and memory problems, and vocabulary placement levels. Along the way, this *Guide* explains the cognitive neuroscience behind each of these reading and learning problems and provides the evidence-based remediation steps that parents can take to help their children experience academic success—and pass their state's standards tests.

Chapter One explains the learning barriers, frequently invisible, that handicap so many bright students. Chapter One also describes my journey developing this program to help my cousin's son Danny—as well as hundreds of other students—identify and eliminate or, at the least, diminish, their reading / learning problems.

Chapter Two reveals how parents can identify their children's specific reading and learning barriers.

Chapter Three shows parents how they can remove, or diminish, critical barriers to reading and learning in their fourth-grade through beginning-college students.

Chapter Four provides suggestions for parents of preschool and early-elementary school children so that they can help their children avoid school failure and frustration through early identification and remediation of likely reading and learning problems. Specifically, Part One of Chapter Four extends this *Guide's* Basic Program to younger students, while Part Two of Chapter Four provides suggestions to educators who might want to institutionalize the Basic Program for their students.

Chapter Five concludes with a discussion of possible environmental causes of what appears to be an ever-increasing number of students who are struggling with attention, memory, visual and auditory dyslexias, and vocabulary problems.

All elements of this *Guide's* Basic Program are based on university, clinical, and foundation research; that is, every component of the Basic Program is evidence-based. Together, these components provide powerful tools for student success, tools that I have experienced when working with hundreds of students in pilot studies and case study investigations.

Please note that although the information presented in this book reflects my extensive learning differences research, along with what I have learned from my students' great success with the Basic Program, no one person or program can successfully eliminate all the possible causes of students' learning difficulties. This Basic Program is designed for students whose learning difficulties are mild to moderate, but not severe. However, even students with severe problems may experience some learning and reading improvement through the information presented herein; this is especially the case if students are seriously affected by Irlen Syndrome.

The Basic Program in no way relieves parents of their responsibility to consult with their children's medical providers to rule out the possibility that their children are experiencing unidentified vision, hearing, or medical problems that may be adversely impacting their learning. Furthermore, parents need to respect any medical advice that they are given and, possibly, seek additional advice from learning specialists. They also need to know that some medical and learning specialists may not be aware of recent cognitive neuroscience research. *A Practical Guide's* Basic Program is supported by cutting-edge cognitive neuroscience research detailing how the brain learns.

This book's recommendations, however, are made without any guarantees for success because, ultimately, parents, teachers, school psychologists, and learning specialists—along with the children themselves—must be responsible for applying the recommendations and suggestions in each individual case. All liability related to the use of this book, therefore, is disclaimed by the author and the publisher. Having made this necessary disclaimer, I will end my "Preface for parents" with the prediction that many more struggling students will join the many students who have already been helped by *A Practical Guide's* Basic Program.

> *Please also note* that the identities of students and colleagues
> have been modified to protect their anonymity.

CHAPTER ONE

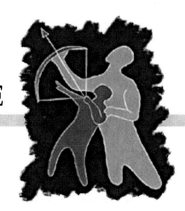

Introduction
How this book will help students succeed

Shoot for the Stars! A Practical Guide for Helping Your Child Achieve Success in School and the Workplace (which I will refer to from now on simply as *A Practical Guide* or the *Guide*) is the culmination of a decades-long journey searching for effective tools to help students struggling with reading and learning. This search began when, as a professor of psychology, I discovered that many bright students are blocked by learning difficulties invisible to their parents and teachers—and often to the students themselves. My search became more urgent when my cousin's son Danny was labeled "learning disabled" despite his obvious intelligence. If my cousin and I had not discovered and corrected the true sources of Danny's learning difficulties, I am certain that Danny's story, along with the stories of my other struggling students, would have ended in academic failure.

> *Note for parents:* Parents eager to get their child started on the path to greater academic success can turn directly to the end of this chapter to find a "Sneak Preview" of this Guide's free Internet assessments and learn about effective reading and learning computer software remediation exercises. Further information about how to set up an individualized brain-building program for their student is presented at the end of Chapters Two and Three.

Over the course of many years, through my research and work with literally thousands of students, I have discovered that nearly all students in the U.S. lack the vocabulary they need for academic success. I also have learned that most students who struggle with reading have problems with attention, working memory, and visual-perceptual or auditory cognitive processing. Most of these students have not been diagnosed with a learning "disability," and my goal in writing *A Practical Guide* is not to so diagnose them. The learning difficulties that I will discuss in this book—namely, Irlen Syndrome visual-perceptual dyslexia, and auditory-processing dyslexia, along with attention deficit—are much more common than parents and teachers realize. I call these reading and learning difficulties "invisible" because they often are not recognized by parents and teachers—or by the students themselves.

In addition, students' learning problems can be present to varying degrees. Students minimally affected may not be diagnosed at all; they struggle alone without ever reaching their true academic potential. Even students' moderate learning difficulties can escape detection. Indeed, I have discovered that many capable students find ways to compensate for their reading and learning difficulties. Unfortunately, the time comes when these students hit their ceiling and reach the grade level where their compensatory strategies begin to fail.

On some level these failing students do realize that they are not fulfilling their true academic potential, and, as a result, most of them suffer from serious test anxiety that only adds to their academic failures. Some of these students may give up on school altogether and drop out. Many students become mental drop-outs before they become physical drop-outs.

Although scientific knowledge about learning problems is still incomplete, educators are aware that American literacy levels are too low, and that too many American students of all ages struggle to read with proficiency. Most educators agree that the number of students with learning problems and below-grade-level reading ability is unacceptably high. Furthermore, educators are learning from new research in the brain sciences that the human brain—throughout the life span—is remarkably "plastic" and able to learn (Beatty, 2001; Leamnson, 2000). Finally, educators have a growing awareness that effective interventions exist and that many of these interventions are in the form of computer software exercises that can "rewire" students' brains and minimize, or eliminate, the brain-based difficulties that prevent them from reading and learning (Posner & Rothbart, 2005; Robertson, 2000; Tallal, 1993).

Based upon cutting-edge scientific research, and strengthened by years of experience helping students succeed, *A Practical Guide* brings to parents effective ways to identify and remediate their children's "invisible" barriers to reading and learning.

In Chapter Two, parents will learn how to identify their children's specific reading and learning barriers. In Chapter Three, parents will learn how to remove, or at least greatly diminish, these specific barriers through simple interventions and computer software exercises that are effective and relatively inexpensive.

Elementary-school and high-school students, as well as beginning college students, have responded enthusiastically to the interventions that I present in this *Guide*. Students in pilot tests of these interventions have gained at least one year in reading grade level with only 24-25 hours of practice over six to eight weeks. Most students have advanced considerably more grade levels, some as many as four, and a few students have gained as many as five grade levels in reading. Students also report enjoyment when reading, whereas previously they had avoided reading altogether. Students report that their physical distress when reading or studying is diminished or entirely eliminated. As a result, reluctant students have become enthusiastic students. Most students report that their grade point averages and test scores have improved.

A minority of students who have severe learning problems may require more extensive professional help than this book can provide. However, *A Practical Guide* also provides helpful resources for parents whose children's learning problems are severe. For example, students with attention problems may benefit from neuropsychiatrist Dr. Daniel Amen's Clinic website (www.amenclinic.com), where students and parents can complete an Attention Deficit Hyperactivity Disorder (ADHD) subtype assessment. After answering questions regarding problematic behaviors adversely impacting learning, Dr. Amen's site supplies helpful information about possible and probable ADHD subtypes along with diet, exercise, nutritional supplements, and medication suggestions. In this way, Dr. Amen's site provides excellent advice that could easily cost hundreds of dollars if provided by a private-practice psychiatrist. Dr. Amen's helpful ADHD books and videos are also available on his website, along with the addresses and contact information of his clinics where diagnostic brain scans and cognitive-behavioral therapy are available.

All of the resources described in this book are evidence-based and supported by scientific research carried out over the past two decades in universities and clinics around the world. Furthermore, this book provides addresses of the best websites where parents can find free assessments to identify their child's specific cognitive and visual-perceptual barriers to reading and learning. If a child is struggling with invisible—that is, difficult-to-identify—handicaps, such as Irlen Syndrome dyslexia, mild or moderate ADHD, or other visual or auditory-processing difficulties, then these free assessment websites will help parents identify their child's specific learning problems. Again, once identified with the assessments provided in Chapter Two, most children's learning difficulties can be decreased, or even eliminated, by the interventions and exercises described in Chapter Three.

By following this *Guide's* suggestions, parents will arm themselves with the information they need to help their child become a more proficient reader and learner. In addition, parents will have the information they need to seek help from appropriate professionals if they discover that their child's problems are severe. Because the effective assessment and remediation resources this book provides are all supported by scientific research and evidence—much new and cutting-edge—I am confident that *A Practical Guide* will help many of our nation's struggling students become competent readers and learners who will pass their state's standards tests.

Parent-to-parent

Raising a child, especially a child who is not working up to his or her potential, is difficult. Parents become frustrated; the child becomes more and more frustrated, and even rebellious, as parents and teachers urge the child to work more and to try harder. Parents and teachers meet and discover their agreement that this child *should* be learning more, *should* be reading on grade level, and *should* be remembering more about the readings. Parents and teachers agree that this child *should* be completing assignments more consistently, paying more attention in class, and in general *should* be progressing more rapidly. Usually, parents and teachers will agree that this child is bright and capable but, for reasons unknown, not keeping up with classmates and not meeting the grade level standards. Sometimes teachers and parents—and more ominously the child—secretly begin to think that maybe this child is not capable, maybe this child is stupid.

Arguments about changing "should" to "is" can generate a series of escalating battles, first between the child and the teacher, then between the child and the parents and, finally, between the parents and the school. With parents, teachers, and children shouldering the added pressures of rising academic standards, and with new state testing requirements under "No Child Left Behind," it's little wonder that tempers flare, fingers of blame point, and the under-achieving child's learning suffers.

As a parent, and especially as a surrogate parent to my cousin's son, I have "been there, done that." I know from personal experience how difficult raising a bright, under-achieving child can be. I also know from years of experience helping my cousin Nan raise her son Danny that even well-intentioned teachers and parents can give up in exasperation when trying to help a child with hidden barriers to learning. Helping Nan raise Danny taught me much about the multiple "invisible" learning problems even bright children can harbor. When I began working with middle-school, high-school, and college students with learning problems, I could apply lessons learned from Danny. Over the past two decades teaching students with hidden barriers to reading and learning, I gained more insight and began to develop programs to identify and remediate my students' problems.

The hidden problems Danny suffered are, I believe, even more prevalent today. When Danny was in school in the 1970s, bright children with Danny's problems often were not properly diagnosed. Children like Danny who struggled with reading and learning were labeled "learning disabled"; in this way they were stigmatized with a label that became a self-fulfilling prophesy. In the 1970s, a few common learning problems had not yet been identified and many helpful interventions were unknown. Today, although much more is known about common barriers to children's reading and learning success, this knowledge is not widespread. Because Danny suffered from many of these problems, I want to share his story with parents.

Danny's story

My cousin Nan confided to me that Danny was hyperactive even before birth. During the last few months of her pregnancy, Nan avoided gatherings where people could stare at her very-pregnant abdomen-in-motion. Danny was making his presence felt and visible before his arrival. Of the two types of hyperactive boys, Danny was more a sweet naïve "Dennis the Menace" than the rather oppositional-defiant "Calvin" of "Calvin and Hobbs" fame. Dark curly hair and big brown eyes, Danny definitely carried the genetic makeup of our Native-American grandfather. Our grandmother was fond of describing her husband as a very active man who would "jump on his horse and ride off in two directions at the same time." Nan and I agreed that this grandpa was one ancestor responsible for Danny's whirlwind energies. On the other side of Nan's family, we located a grandmother who exhibited the inconsistent mental habits and nervous energy that we thought contributed to Danny's double genetic dose of attention problems.

Because Danny was bright, his dyslexia showed up mainly in low spelling scores, a dislike of reading, especially aloud, and a great reluctance to write book reports. With my and Nan's tutoring help and encouragement, Danny compensated well, and

Nan's frequent presence at teachers' "conferences" diminished. When Danny was in senior high, Nan returned from work late one afternoon and was greeted by an excited Danny. "Mom," Danny exclaimed, "I saw a TV program on Attention Deficit Hyperactivity Disorder where a kid was bouncing around the classroom just like I did in grammar school. Maybe I don't have dyslexia, maybe I have ADHD!" To Nan, this self-diagnosis was a revelation that rang true. Nan knew, however, that Danny did have many characteristics of dyslexia. She had taken Danny for diagnosis to Dr. Harold Solan, a well-known ophthalmologist whose dyslexia treatments involved eye exercises, and she also had received advice from special education teachers whose ideas about helping dyslexics involved extra reading, especially reading aloud.

In college Danny was still struggling to work up to his considerable potential. That was in the eighties when Helen Irlen's work with dyslexics was becoming known. Helen Irlen, a learning disability specialist, school psychologist, and educational therapist, had discovered that some dyslexics suffered from a little-understood problem she called Scotopic Sensitivity Syndrome (SSS). SSS, now called Irlen Syndrome, can cause many learning problems, including symptoms of dyslexia. Irlen Syndrome, for example, can cause students to misread words and to misunderstand what is read. In addition, Irlen Syndrome can cause symptoms of attention deficit, such as an inability to stay on task for very long. Moreover, students like Danny—who was severely affected by Irlen Syndrome—can develop headaches and stomachaches, and become very fatigued when reading. Little wonder that as a result these students avoid reading!

Naturally bright, Danny had been compensating for his learning difficulties with Nan's and my tutoring help. However, like many children with learning difficulties, Danny, we discovered, had more than one genetic "glitch." Danny was struggling with multiple learning problems: His hyperactivity, inattention, impulsivity, coupled with his lack of follow-through described his ADHD; his visual-motor and visual-perceptual problems reflected symptoms of Irlen Syndrome dyslexia. As he advanced in school and encountered increasing academic challenges, Danny began to hit his ceiling as his ability to compensate began to fail him. Nan and I needed help helping

Danny, but the psychologist at his college could offer no suggestions: He tested Danny and reported that he was a gifted student who obviously suffered from a neurotic mother and aunt!

Luckily for Danny, Nan, and me, an article about the Irlen Method had just appeared in a local newspaper. Although Danny had been helped by Dr. Harold Solan's visual-training exercises some years before, and his eye muscle weaknesses had been corrected, he was still experiencing several difficulties when reading—and in college he was expected to read more than ever before. Because Danny's symptoms of fatigue when reading, his losing his place, and his having to reread frequently fit the symptoms described for Irlen Syndrome dyslexia, we decided to have Danny tested at Helen Irlen's International Headquarters in Long Beach, California. We discovered that Danny indeed was seriously affected by Irlen Syndrome. When he was supplied with reading lenses tinted in the color that best alleviated his symptoms, Danny's fatigue when reading disappeared and his reading comprehension improved enormously.

Many experts now agree that Irlen Syndrome accounts for one type of dyslexia, and they agree that students seriously affected can also experience problems that mimic ADHD, for example, restlessness and inattention when reading. Of course, Irlen Syndrome can co-exist with ADHD and other dyslexias. Such was the case with Danny who was discovered to also have an auditory-processing difficulty that made it difficult for him to process material he heard when the material was rapidly presented. This auditory-processing difficulty is associated with a common type of dyslexia and will be explained in greater detail later. Nan and I, along with the expert help of other learning specialists, including nutritionists and neuropsychiatrists at Dr. Daniel Amen's Newport Beach Clinic, have provided Danny with the interventions he needed to complete a demanding Bachelor's Program in the University of California system. Now Danny has entered the professional world of work and, although he still has to work a bit harder than other intellectually gifted persons, he has accomplished a great deal despite his many genetic glitches.

Danny certainly is exceptional in his intellectual gifts and in the number of problems he had to overcome. Danny is, however, by no means unusual. Many of the students I have worked with over the years also have experienced multiple learning difficulties rooted in problematic genetics. The assessments and remediation interventions that this *Guide* presents, along with the brain-building exercises I recommend, have helped Danny and my students, and they can provide parents with the knowledge they need to identify and decrease, or even eliminate, their children's learning problems.

My students' stories

After completing an interdisciplinary doctorate in psychology and social theory at the University of California, Irvine, I began teaching graduate school in Irvine for Pepperdine University's Graduate School of Education and Psychology and for United States International University. To my surprise, I found that even in graduate school some students struggled with reading and learning problems. Because I was teaching masters- and doctoral-level students in clinical psychology programs, students would ask me for advice, not only in regard to their studies, but also with respect to their personal struggles with their children, spouses, and parents. From their stories, I began to gain insight into the intergenerational problems Irlen Syndrome and auditory-processing dyslexias, combined with attention deficit, can cause. As I counseled these students, I would learn that the reading and learning difficulties of a husband were now manifesting themselves in a child's similar difficulties. One woman student came to me for advice regarding juggling her studies with the problems posed by her hyperactive son and ADHD husband; her husband demonstrated no patience with their son, nor did he understand her difficulties in completing her graduate school assignments while mediating family disputes.

I was able to reassure my student that many family conflicts occurred between family members sharing the same genetic problems. For example, Nan's father was *very* severely affected by ADHD; this grandpa had little tolerance for Danny's loud voice and rambunctious behaviors that, he complained, "get on my nerves." In addition,

I could refer my students to learning and behavior modification resources that had helped Danny cope academically and socially.

Often students would become aware of the intergenerational aspects of learning problems when discussing their children's learning difficulties with me. They would suddenly recognize that they themselves, or another family member, had been struggling with the same problems when learning to read. Students who would enter my office to tearfully describe their children's learning problems, and sometimes their own, would leave smiling because relieved of feelings of guilt and helplessness. They would leave understanding that many family conflicts result from difficult genetics and are not their fault. They also would leave armed with knowledge about learning differences and about the resources available for understanding and alleviating the academic failures and low self-esteem issues that feed many family conflicts.

My insights into students' barriers to learning deepened dramatically when I accepted a full-time teaching assignment at a Central Washington State college. Here my students' family conflicts and struggles to complete degrees were compounded by rural isolation, poverty or working-class status, demanding work schedules in minimum-wage jobs, histories of domestic abuse, chemical dependency, divorce and single parenthood. For over a third of my students, English was a second language. Approximately 60 percent of my students were women and about 30 percent were older, non-traditional college students, many returning to school after having sustained on-the-job injuries—or they were returning as "welfare-to-work" single parents.

By the end of my first quarter teaching I had detected one major problem that all of my college students shared whether they were English-language learners, older students, or young high-achieving high school students: All of my students, almost without exception, lacked a college-level vocabulary. When I inquired of English Department colleagues why the college wasn't teaching vocabulary, a seasoned—and excellent—older colleague informed me that she had taught a vocabulary course that had been discontinued some years earlier. "Students enjoyed my course," she noted, "I taught them word families and dictionary skills that students today are sorely lacking." This colleague, now nearing retirement, informed me that she had noticed a serious decline in her students' English-language skills 20 years ago. "I knew that this decline would continue and even worsen," she told me, "because the students of 20 years ago had very poor skills, and they have become the elementary and high-school teachers of present-day college students." Most of my college colleagues would agree that their students are entering college more and more unprepared for college work, but most of them apparently are not aware of how greatly their students are suffering from a lack of word power.

My awareness of this critical student deficit increased over the course of my first year as students came to me during multiple choice exams to ask me to provide synonyms for words such as "precede," "autocratic," and "accomplished." Most of my students who were failing these exams were failing simply because they were lacking in word power. I soon came to recognize that many young students, even those from more affluent family backgrounds, were not aware of the degree to which their impoverished vocabularies were limiting them.

Some older students were, however, aware of their lack. For example, one older female student acutely felt her vocabulary deficiencies. A former farmer's wife, plump and matronly, her hair graying, this student approached me one day after class and pleaded with me to help her. "My mother only had a third-grade education," she told me. "I've worked most of my life on a farm. What can I do to stay in school and succeed? *I just don't have the words to understand your lectures or the textbook.*" Her tone was anguished, and in that moment I knew that she spoke for nearly all of my students, female and male, of all ages and ethnicities. Her simple phrase, *"I just don't have the words,"* has echoed in my mind ever since. It was then that I resolved to find a way to increase students' vocabulary levels.

To my surprise, I met with resistance from a few of my younger English Department colleagues who told me when I suggested reinstituting a vocabulary-building course,

"Oh, we do teach vocabulary in our developmental English courses," one colleague reassured me, "but we insist on teaching vocabulary in context." Of course, if students had to learn all vocabulary words and other facts "in context," the process would be so slow that cultural knowledge could never be transmitted to succeeding generations! I again was surprised shortly thereafter when discussing our students' academic needs with another young English Department colleague. I mentioned that working-class mothers were more apt to *show* their children how to do something rather than *tell* them how to do something. "Most of our students come from families struggling economically and, therefore, are better kinesthetic learners and visual learners," I said, "than lecture-only learners. Typically, they are *shown* and not *told* how to do something. Typically, our students from poverty-level and working-class families are not exposed much to spoken language, either through verbal interactions with parents or by being read to."

My young colleague, who had been listening thoughtfully, suddenly exclaimed as if she had just understood something entirely foreign to her, "You mean to tell me that most of our entering college students do not have the vocabulary required to access our college texts!" she exclaimed. To me, my colleague's outburst was a revelation because I could not believe that someone who had been teaching developmental and beginning English college courses for several years had not recognized one of our students' most critical deficiencies.

Indeed, more and more I saw that impoverished vocabularies are not limited only to students from economically-deprived families. I began to observe that even my more economically-privileged white students' vocabularies were also impoverished. Supporting my observations was the previously mentioned Gallup survey conducted in 1950 that found that the average American fourteen-year-old's vocabulary contained 25,000 words. When Gallup reran the survey in 1999, they discovered that the average 14-year-old's vocabulary had dropped to 10,000 words (Worldwatch Institute, 2000). A researcher at the vocabulary-building software company I recommend told me that the decline in average vocabulary continues to this day. Reading experts have noted that children who fall behind in vocabulary, for whatever reason, may never catch up, and that the fewer the vocabulary words children know, the poorer is their reading comprehension and academic achievement (Chall & Jacobs, 2003).

"Having the words," then, is the indispensable foundation for understanding what is read and heard. In fact, in an article entitled, "The Early Catastrophe," developmental psychology researchers Professors Betty Hart and Todd Risley (2003) have discovered a "30 million word gap by age 3" in most poverty-level children when compared with children from professional-level families. Hart and Risley found that children from families in higher income brackets are exposed to more frequent and complex language in conversation and books. Their extensive research finds that poverty-level children have heard 30 million fewer words during their first few years of life than children from professional families (Allen & Sethi, 2004; Hart, & Risley, 2003).

Therefore, the foundation of this book's reading / learning program is the best vocabulary-building software program on the market, namely, WordSmart, a program based on 70 years of research linking individuals' word knowledge, that is, their vocabulary levels, to their levels of professional accomplishment in an increasingly competitive job market.

I knew, however, that my students of diverse ages and ethnicities were hindered academically by more than just poor vocabularies. As I began this new college teaching assignment, I also began to notice the large numbers of students who had symptoms of attention deficit and whose reading and writing clearly reflected problems of dyslexia.

Many students had trouble staying focused and paying attention in class. Many of them would ask to speak with me after class and tell me that they had been diagnosed with ADHD; some had even been labeled "retarded" in elementary school because of their learning problems. During one unforgettable quarter, I had nine of my *Introduction to Psychology* class's 27 students speak with me privately and ask me if they could choose the topic of ADHD for their research paper, a summary of which they would also present orally to their classmates. Each of these students shyly admitted in turn that they had been diagnosed with ADHD.

Naturally I was pleased to approve my students' choice of ADHD as a research topic, and I asked them if they would like to present their research findings as a group to the rest of the class. The students willingly agreed, and they appeared especially eager to work with classmates who were struggling with the same learning problem. On the day these nine students presented their findings, they sat at desks lined up in front of the class; each of the nine competently presented the particular aspect of ADHD that they had chosen to research. As well-socialized ADHD individuals, my students' appearance above the desks was calm and controlled; below the desks, their ADHD nervous systems were manifesting in continuously swinging legs as if all nine were performing in unison a subtle French cancan!

These students and their classmates learned much from their ADHD research projects, as do the many dyslexic students I teach who also are eager to research and share information about their learning difficulties. I am always gratified when students have the courage to come to me after class and tell me that they have been diagnosed with a learning difference. Note that I prefer the term, "difference," to the term, "disability," because a "learning difference" label is, in my opinion, a more accurate designation and less likely to set students up for failure than labeling them with a "learning disability." Students gain the courage to confide in me, I believe, because I always explain what researchers in cognitive psychology know to be true, namely, that having one or more learning difficulties does not a stupid student make.

Unfortunately, there is much confusion among the general public, in the minds of parents, and even in the minds of some educators regarding the abilities of students with visual-perceptual (Irlen Syndrome) and auditory-processing dyslexia and ADHD. Most individuals with these problems can become proficient readers, thinkers, and learners. *A Practical Guide* will show parents how to help their children improve and succeed academically and, eventually, in the workplace. In fact, learning specialists have found that there are many reasons why students struggle academically—and stupidity is not one of these reasons. Higher-level reasoning and creativity are most often intact in these students; once their specific learning problems are identified and remediated, most students can soar to higher levels of accomplishment (Hallowell & Ratey, 1994; Shaywitz, 2003; Sternberg & Grigorenko, 1999).

Recognizing the high percentage of my college students who struggle with reading and learning, and the low self-esteem and high degree of test anxiety that result, I emphasize to all my students that having learning differences does not mean they are stupid or incapable of learning. I tell them about the author of their *Introduction to Psychology* textbook, the eminent Prof. Robert Sternberg, and I recount how he struggled as a young student with test anxiety and lower-than-expected IQ scores. I tell students how Prof. Sternberg identified his own area of cognitive weakness and how he compensated for this relative weakness, eliminated his test anxiety, and raised his IQ scores. I give students the good news that IQ scores are not written in stone—or on their foreheads. My students are always relieved to learn that they should not permit relatively low IQ scores to discourage them because, I explain, human brains are malleable, and students' learning problems can be identified and remediated. When I tell students about the many success stories I have witnessed, these students gain the motivation they need to discover and eliminate their hidden barriers so they, too, can experience greater academic success (Begley, S., 1996; Neisser, 1998).

At the end of my lecture to students about intelligence and IQ scores, students often stay after class to tell me their stories. These student stories have given me insight into why students do not succeed in school and why they may continue their patterns of failure in their jobs and relationships. Some students report having been labeled "learning disabled," or even "retarded," in elementary school. I admire the courage of these students who somehow have managed to overcome such negative labels and enter college. One of these students told me that she recognized, despite the label "retarded," that she had ability. She studied learning difficulties and diagnosed herself with ADHD and dyslexia shortly after her son was diagnosed with ADHD and dyslexia. His IQ was very high, she told me, and despite his problems with reading, he was tutoring high school students in math while still in middle school.

Another student came to me after class to tell me that she thought she might be dyslexic because she had been so diagnosed in elementary school. However, she told me that her mother had rejected this diagnosis, and she confided that "My mom told the teacher that I was too smart to be dyslexic." After hearing my lecture on learning differences and intelligence, this student told me that she now realizes that she probably is dyslexic—*and* intelligent! She told me that now her task is to identify exactly what type of dyslexia she has and discover how to remediate and diminish her reading and writing problems. This student's story is among the many student stories that have inspired my research, as well as the development of this book's Basic Program for assessment and remediation of the most common barriers keeping students from realizing their full academic potential.

Although having one-third of my students in one class exhibiting ADHD symptoms was rather extreme, as the following years unfolded I found that almost every class I taught at this college would contain at least one, and usually several students, some diagnosed and some not diagnosed, with ADHD and / or dyslexia behaviors. Therefore, combining my knowledge of Danny's multiple learning difficulties, including ADHD and dyslexia, with knowledge I was gaining from my rural college students' stories, I decided to run a small study to discover the extent to which students harbored problems with attention deficits. Parents can see the results of my small study on Graph A at the end of this chapter (page 39).

Using a standard ADD questionnaire, this study was stratified by gender and ethnicity. The results show that about half of the self-selected student sample probably, or possibly, harbors some degree of attention deficit. Although this percentage might appear too high, my 13 years of experience with students at this rural college have revealed the existence of just such high percentages of students with serious barriers to learning. Widespread poverty, drug and alcohol addictions, and low literacy rates in parental and student generations easily provide multiple overlapping explanations for students' academic achievement difficulties (Evans, 2004).

Early program results

As in most studies conducted in educational settings where students are asked but not forced to provide answers to standard questionnaires, there is an unavoidable "self-selection" bias. I was not interested in attaching a negative label (for example, "ADD" or "ADHD") to students, but instead I wanted to discover ways to help students pay attention and learn. Therefore, I presented my research studies to students as investigations into how they learn best. Parents can see from the results of my ADD survey that over half of this sample of entering students who agreed to complete my survey does struggle with some degree of ADD or ADHD. When I would speak to my college colleagues about the high numbers of our students who were struggling with some degree of attention deficit and / or dyslexia, at first these colleagues did not recognize the symptoms and behaviors, and they would tell me that I was exaggerating.

Again, I must emphasize that a student struggling with attention or dyslexia problems often is not easily identified. Many, if not most, students are compensating more or less successfully for their problems. Most do not fit neatly into simple black or white, either / or, categories. Attention deficits and visual-perceptual or auditory processing dyslexias exist on a spectrum from very mild to very severe. As Dr. Isabelle Rapin (2002) states in her essay on Thomas Sowell's, *The Einstein Syndrome*, normality has "fuzzy margins" at its edges and "a wide range of severity." Dr. Rapin goes on to state that "there is no crisp partition between normalcy and disorder, and between disorders with different names yet shared features, even when there is no controversy regarding the identification of prototypic exemplars" (p. 49). Researchers in the cognitive neurosciences are only beginning to scratch the surface of the many interacting genetic and environmental causes of learning "differences." Meanwhile, students, along with parents and teachers, struggle to find solutions.

Interestingly, by the end of my second year teaching at this rural college, some of my "doubting Thomas" colleagues began admitting, "You are right!" when I would refer to our college's many ADHD and dyslexia-affected students. "They indeed are everywhere!" one colleague exclaimed. When I told a college administrator that nearly half of our students harbored some learning differences, I was interested to hear him respond that "Dr. Morrow, I believe that *more* than half of our students have learning disabilities." Of course, I did believe that more than half of our students had learning differences which were causing them to fall short of their learning potential. In fact, the more I learned about student diversity in learning, the more I agreed with Dr. Mel Levine's assertions that students do have "all kinds of minds" (Levine, 1999). I therefore resolved to continue my observations and surveys of student learning difficulties with the goal of developing programs that would help these different minds achieve greater academic proficiency.

I began working with my colleagues in local elementary schools; there I learned that growing problems of chemical dependency in our area were increasing the number of elementary school students with learning problems caused by parents' alcohol and drug addictions. Unfortunately, some students' learning problems can be attributed to maternal, and even paternal, chemical addictions that have damaged sperm and the child's developing brain before birth. Most parents are aware of this possibility and try to refrain from using drugs, drinking alcohol, and smoking when they decide to conceive a child. A few parents, regrettably, are not aware—or, if aware of the danger to their unborn child, are unable to stop ingesting harmful substances.

However, most learning difficulties like ADHD and various dyslexias have genetic origins. Research studies over the past two decades have begun to locate the genes responsible for some learning problems, and to document that these problems do tend to run in families (Robinson, G. L., 1997; Schumacher et al., 2006). Further complicating the identification of causes for learning problems is the well-documented fact that genetically-caused chemical imbalances in the brain can predispose individuals to chemical addictions. These individuals often attempt to self-medicate their ADHD or dyslexia with alcohol, drugs, and by smoking.

Despite the unsolved difficulties in identifying specific learning problems, and despite the causal complexity that accompanies these learning problems, *A Practical Guide* brings good news to parents, even those parents who may have unwittingly consumed drugs and other toxic chemicals when conceiving and carrying a child. The recent research inspiring this book provides evidence that unless students' brain damage is severe (and perhaps even then), most students' brains can be improved by means of the remediations provided in Chapter Three. Neuroscience research over the past decade reveals that human brains, even adult brains, are "plastic"—meaning malleable—and, therefore, capable of being rewired if students are provided with exercises targeted to their specific areas of weakness (Kleinfeld & Wescott, 1993). These research findings offer hope for all students who apply themselves to improving their identified specific learning problems, an identification task made easier by this *Guide's* Chapter Two.

Developing the Basic Program

After observing the large proportion of my college students with impoverished vocabularies, attention problems, and various degrees and types of dyslexia, I began to work with colleagues to develop programs that would identify and remediate these problems. One of my colleagues had developed a computerized assessment program based on Wechsler IQ subtests. This program identified students' visual and / or auditory sequencing problems, their visual and / or auditory memory problems, and their problems with comprehension. Students' vocabulary levels, and their visual-motor memory and visual-motor learning abilities also were assessed.

Once their specific learning problems were found, students were successfully remediated with a very effective program of computer software exercises that I developed. The program worked so well that my college was paid by Washington State's Department of Social and Health Services to improve the reading, learning, and workforce performance of their clients enrolled in the State's Welfare-to-Work initiative. I also institutionalized the program for my college's students, as well as at a nearby federal Job Corps school. At all of these locations, this program met with enthusiastic support from students whose learning abilities were improving, as evidenced by post-program reassessments and teachers' reports.

One teacher at the Job Corps school reported that students were distressed when the computer lab running these remediation exercises closed for repairs. Students were eager to continue doing their assigned brain-building exercises because they found these exercises fun. Further, they reported that they could actually sense their improved cognitive functioning. Another teacher at this school reported that student scores on their term-ending "Test of Adult Basic Education" (TABE) had greatly improved, especially in reading and math. In fact, she told me that "students' scores are up in all subjects." I was pleased and encouraged by these reports, especially given that this Job Corps school served at-risk 16- to 24-year-old school drop-outs, many of whom were street kids suffering from years of abuse, neglect, and chemical dependency.

Unfortunately, as so often happens, even with successful programs, Washington State funding for the programs ran out, and my college was forced to shut the program down. However, with the insight and knowledge I had gained, I was convinced that an even better reading enhancement and learning program could be developed. I had noticed that when some student subtest scores, specifically, visual-motor learning and visual-motor memory were low, students' scores on a screening questionnaire for visual-perceptual dyslexia were usually quite high. Irlen Syndrome causes visual-perceptual problems that may lead to debilitating physical symptoms and many other reading and learning problems. Students develop headaches, and even migraines, when reading or doing computer work, and they complain of fatigue, stomachaches, muscle tension, and an inability to stay focused on their work. As with other types of dyslexia, students also complain about losing their place when reading, about misreading, about not comprehending or remembering what they read, and about slow laborious reading where the words often appear to move about on the page or to blur and even disappear.

More than a decade prior to my present teaching assignment in Washington State, I had read about Helen Irlen's work with learning-disabled students and her discovery that many of her students responded well to having colored transparencies placed over their reading material. I remembered that Danny had been found to have Irlen Syndrome, had been tested at Helen Irlen's Long Beach International Headquarters, and had responded well to the Irlen intervention of appropriately-tinted lenses. Now, with the permission of Helen Irlen, I began to assess my students to discover how many might be affected by Irlen Syndrome. With the help of a colleague who is our college's best qualified reading instructor, I used the Irlen "Reading Strategies Questionnaire" and asked a large number of students in reading and social science courses to respond. The results shown in Graph B (pages 40-41) at the end of this chapter revealed that upwards of 40 percent of our students would benefit from further screening and, most probably, would benefit from appropriately-colored transparencies placed over material when they read or over their computer screens. Of this 40 percent, many would further benefit if provided with appropriately-tinted lenses.

In addition, I had continued to survey my students for over a decade to discover other learning problems they struggled to overcome. Almost all of my struggling students, as well as my colleagues' struggling students, complained of working-memory problems, particularly in the auditory-learning modality. My students, like so many across this country, quite simply are not good lecture-only learners. I documented these student problems in a number of courses, as well as more informally, by asking students to indicate their favorite way to learn—visually, auditorily, kinesthetically (hands-on)—by a show of hands. The results of my more formal documentation of students' favorite way(s) to learn is shown at the end of this chapter's Graph C (page 42).

As can readily be seen from Graph C, most of my college's students are not good auditory, lecture-only, learners. In fact, my reading instructor colleague recently attended a national reading conference where she learned that across the U.S., more than 90 percent of American students now are reported to be kinesthetic, hands-on, learners. Few learn well without hands-on and / or visual support when facts and concepts are presented. Furthermore, recent research, discussed in more detail in Chapter Two, reports that attention deficits and dyslexias, including Irlen Syndrome, are much more prevalent than parents and educators realize (Amen, 2005; Irvine, 2005; Shaywitz, 2003).

Many bright students who are affected by attention deficit, dyslexia, and / or Irlen Syndrome, but not severely affected, are compensating, as was Danny with Nan's and my help. However, even bright students will fall far short of their academic and professional potential if not helped by the cutting-edge research presented in this *Guide*. Sadly, most struggling students have not had their specific learning problems uncovered precisely because they are compensating so well—that is, until they hit their ceiling when they can no longer function at grade level. Some students, like so many of my beginning college students, do not begin to fail until they enter college where the reading and learning demands accelerate dramatically over what most of them had experienced in high school.

Most struggling students, unlike Danny, do not have a relative who understands and has made a specialty of studying learning problems. Most struggling students are harboring unidentified learning difficulties and, unlike Danny's case, these difficulties remain invisible to parents, teachers, and to the students themselves. Of course, the more severe a student's learning problem is, the earlier that student will begin to fail. Early failure, however, is no guarantee that the appropriate assessments and interventions will be forthcoming. All too often, these failing students are labeled "learning disabled" and relegated to resource rooms where their true problems remain unremediated and the label "disabled" becomes a self-fulfilling prophesy (Catone & Brady, 2005).

The final difficulty that I have observed over and over again in struggling students is severe test anxiety. When reading and learning difficulties have not been properly diagnosed and remediated, students realize that they are, for reasons unknown to them, not working up to their full potential. The harder they try, the more stress they experience, and the more stress hormones erase their memory banks when they confront an important exam. My experience with such students has shown that once they realize that their reading and learning problems are not caused by stupidity, but are caused by a specific deficit, they begin to relax and release themselves from much stress-induced anxiety. As their learning difficulties are eased by the effective interventions and exercises described in Chapter Three, students' self-confidence and self-esteem improve and much of their test anxiety dissipates.

Basic Program overview

One of this *Guide*'s first steps towards helping struggling students is to discover whether Irlen Syndrome is present. Identifying and remediating students for Irlen Syndrome is an essential early step because other assessments will not be as accurate, nor will the other remediation steps be as effective if Irlen Syndrome is present, but remains unremediated. If a student has this visual-perceptual dyslexia, a problem that optometrists and most ophthalmologists are not trained to detect, intervention with colored transparencies or tinted lenses can bring about major improvements in reading, the basis for all learning. Improvements can also occur in students' memory and attention abilities.

For those students severely affected by Irlen Syndrome, the improvement can appear almost miraculous. For example, one 18-year-old Job Corps student who was reading on a second or third-grade level was provided by my Irlen screener with the appropriately-colored transparency. Immediately this student exclaimed, "I can read! I can read!" and he asked if he could run to demonstrate his new proficiency to all of his teachers. If this example appears exaggerated, I can assure parents that I have experienced many similar incidents with students. And, I should also mention that

I, too, have Irlen Syndrome and can testify that even for someone like myself who is only moderately impacted, there is dramatic improvement in my ability to read without fatigue for hours when wearing my tinted lenses. I am not as affected by Irlen Syndrome as Danny, but I do share our family's genetic glitch.

This *Guide*'s next steps involve identifying whether students have problems with attention, memory, vocabulary and other cognitive processes. As parents read Chapter Two, "How to identify hidden barriers to reading and learning," they will learn about the free Internet websites where they can access the assessments that will help them identify these hidden barriers. In addition, they will learn about exciting new cognitive neuroscience research that supports each of the interventions this book recommends. Especially exciting is the research using brain scans of individuals with various learning problems. These scans provide evidence that Irlen Method interventions change for the better the brains of students with Irlen Syndrome. As previously described, these brain-improving Irlen interventions consist quite simply of appropriately-colored transparent reading material overlays or lenses tinted in a color appropriate for the individual student. These colored transparencies are placed over reading materials, and they can also be placed over a computer screen to mute the glare and high contrast that impedes Irlen Syndrome students' reading fluency and comprehension. (In addition, as needed by the individual student, the computer screen's background, brightness, and / or text can be modified using the computer's operating system.)

Other exciting research studies involving remediation of attention deficits are emerging from the laboratory of University of Oregon's Prof. Michael Posner and will be discussed further in Chapter Three. Again, all of the assessments and interventions parents will encounter in Chapters Two and Three are abundantly supported by research conducted in universities, clinics, and laboratories in the U.S. and abroad. These effective assessments and interventions are the foundation for *A Practical Guide*'s Basic Program. By providing their children with this Basic Program, parents will improve their children's reading and learning and, especially, help their children who are struggling academically and in danger of failing their state's standards tests.

My earlier program had been used with great success by my college, and at a Job Corps school, for nearly five years. I have spent the past several summers locating and testing the Basic Program's evidence-based assessments and remediations. Pilot studies carried out with beginning college students and with middle-school age students have demonstrated that this *Guide*'s combined brain-building exercises can remove, or at least reduce, most students' specific reading and learning difficulties while raising their reading grade level at least one year with 24-25 hours of practice over six to eight weeks. Most students in my pilot studies gained several years in reading level and experienced improved grades and test scores. Each of the suggested interventions is evidence-based, and the combination of all of these suggested interventions, therefore, work together to effectively boost students' brain power and their ability to succeed academically.

In summary, Chapter Two will teach parents how to locate the free Internet assessments that will help them identify their children's specific learning difficulties. Chapters Three and Four will show parents how to set up an effective program of remediation to raise their children's reading level and learning abilities. Chapter Three presents the basic intervention program for children in grades four through adult. Chapter Four presents modifications of the basic intervention program with suggestions for preschool and early elementary school-age students. Chapter Five will conclude by discussing additional ways to help students pass the state standards tests, including simple nutritional and lifestyle interventions.

Recognizing students' best learning style is important, but children who apply the Basic Program will increase the ways in which they can access knowledge. These students will have enlarged their learning style capabilities. In short, *A Practical Guide* provides comprehensive, simple, inexpensive, and effective paths for students' academic—and eventual workplace—success.

Sneak Preview of the Program

For parents who are eager to start their Internet search to identify their children's possible learning difficulties, I summarize below the free Internet websites that parents can begin to explore.

Assessments

Step 1: Test Anxiety website: www.wwcc.edu/student_services/online_adv/success/ test_test.cfm. Parents can find Walla Walla Community College's helpful test anxiety questionnaire (along with useful study skills information) by typing this Internet address on their search engine. By reading with their children questions regarding test anxiety, parents can discover the extent to which test anxiety may be adversely affecting their children's academic achievement. Parents should remember that most students who are experiencing severe test anxiety and / or school phobias probably are harboring invisible stumbling blocks that this *Guide*'s Basic Program may alleviate. Once their children's stumbling blocks are identified and remediated, their children's test anxiety should be greatly alleviated as well. In addition, this website's learning styles and study skills assessments will provide clues for parents regarding their children's areas of strength and weakness, along with study strategies for their children once their learning problems have been remediated.

Step 2: Irlen Syndrome website: www.irlen.com. Parents can take the free Irlen Syndrome assessment questionnaire for their children—or with them—and discover if their children have Irlen Syndrome.

Step 3: Attention Deficit website: www.brainplace.com/SPECT (or, www.amenclinic. com). The Brainplace address is Dr. Amen's brain imaging information and resources site. Once at this site, parents should click on "Amen clinics" and then scroll down and click on "Amen Brain System Test." When parents access Dr. Amen's Brain System Test, they can take this free ADD subtype assessment for their children—or with them, depending upon the children's ages—and discover if their children probably, or possibly, have a type of attention deficit adversely impacting their learning ability. Parents will be provided with valuable information regarding diet, supplements, exercise, and medication to treat each ADD subtype.

Step 4: Memory / Attention website: www.parrotsoftware.com. Parents can answer for—or with—their children Parrot Software's free 30-question communication survey. Parents need not be discouraged by Parrot Software's online description stating that these programs "are designed to help people who suffer from speech and communication problems caused by stroke, Alzheimer's, or other forms of brain injury." Parrot Software programs are used in many schools and colleges in the U.S. and around the world to help students of all ages remediate problems with memory, attention, and reasoning skills.

My experience working with students of all ages who have learning difficulties has taught me that starting with remediation for Irlen Syndrome, as needed, and then remediating students' problems with memory, attention, and vocabulary deficiencies constitutes a powerful reading / learning approach for most students who struggle with reading and learning. Once parents have applied all of the Basic Program's Steps, they may want to revisit Parrot Software to identify and remediate other specific cognitive-processing problems that their children are exhibiting.

Step 5: Vocabulary-building website: www.wordsmart.com. Parents can learn about the fastest and most effective way to assess and remediate their children's vocabulary deficiencies on this website. Students from age eight through adult may take the WordSmart challenge for level-of-difficulty placement in this fun vocabulary-building program. Younger students may benefit most from WordSmart's excellent phonics program.

Remediation

The following steps are for parents eager to begin remediating their children's learning problems. *(Note: For more details about assessment and remediation, see Chapters Two and Three.)*

Step 1: Parents can locate a qualified Irlen screener at www.irlen.com. This screener can help parents find the most effective colored transparency to eliminate symptoms associated with Irlen Syndrome. These symptoms may constitute the most significant barriers preventing their children's success in learning to read. Because many children with reading or learning problems have more than one significant stumbling block, parents need to assess their children for each of the above common problems and then remediate these problems as needed.

Step 2: Parents can help their children with auditory-processing dyslexia by obtaining the inexpensive software program called Earobics at the appropriate level. Earobics can be found online at www.earobics.com.

Step 3: Parents can improve their children's attention problems by accessing www.parrotsoftware.com and obtaining the inexpensive attention-building software program "Hierarchical Attention Training."

Step 4: Parents can improve their children's visual and auditory memory problems by accessing www.parrotsoftware.com and obtaining the memory-building software program "Visual and Auditory Memory Span." Also helpful at www.parrotsoftware.com for improving children's listening skills, memory, and attention is the software program, "Word Memory and Discrimination."

Step 5: Parents can improve their children's vocabulary levels with the entertaining and very effective vocabulary-building computer software exercises available at www.wordsmart.com. (Again, for younger children, WordSmart's phonics program is excellent.)

What's ahead

Chapters Two and Three present the research evidence supporting the choice of these specific abilities—namely, memory, attention, and vocabulary—for assessment and remediation, along with more detailed information regarding the identification and remediation of visual-perceptual and auditory-processing dyslexias.

Besides free assessments, these websites also provide remediation information, as well as information regarding other interventions. Chapter Two presents detailed information regarding the use of these websites to identify students' specific learning difficulties, while Chapter Three presents detailed information regarding the best software exercises to remediate these now-identified learning problems. The suggested Basic Program for the most common learning problems can be found at the end of Chapter Three. Chapter Four extends this Basic Program with suggestions for younger children and for educators wishing to institutionalize the Basic Program. Chapter Five concludes with information about important further steps that parents can take to ensure their children's academic success.

> *Note that Appendixes A through B[4] are designed to help parents and older students set up an individual remediation plan [IRP] that will focus on eliminating the specific cognitive-processing problems of each student.*

Suggested reading

Irlen, Helen (2005): *Reading by the colors: Overcoming dyslexia and other reading disabilities through the Irlen method* is Helen Irlen's seminal presentation of Irlen Syndrome, its prevalence, adverse impact on students' reading and learning, and how parents can eliminate the problems this syndrome causes.

Wolfe, Patricia (2001): *Brain matters: Translating research into classroom practice* presents the new cognitive neuroscience understandings about how the brain learns, and can be rewired and effectively taught. This book is simply written and an excellent resource for teachers and those parents who want a deeper understanding of learning and the brain.

Amen, Daniel, M.D. (1998): *Change your brain, Change your life* is neuropsychiatrist Dr. Amen's best-seller that provides amazingly effective prescriptions for solving many students' (and their parents') brain-based problems, including ADHD, anger, anxiety, and depression.

Graph A

ADD Level %

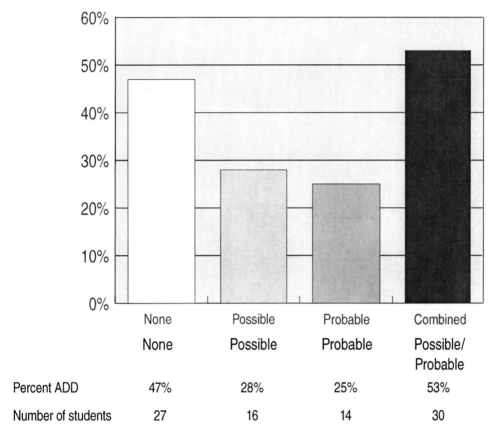

	None None	Possible Possible	Probable Probable	Combined Possible/ Probable
Percent ADD	47%	28%	25%	53%
Number of students	27	16	14	30

The above graph shows the results of my Reading Enhancement & Computerized Learning Program assessment of entering college students (fall 1996). A standard Adult ADD Questionnaire (Brown) instrument was used. My objective was not to label students with attention deficit disorder but to gather information regarding the extent to which entering college students (self-selected sample of 57 students stratified by gender and ethnicity) were struggling to some degree with maintaining their focus and following through on their plans and objectives. This study indicated that a high percentage of entering students at my college might benefit from attention-strengthening exercises.

Graph B

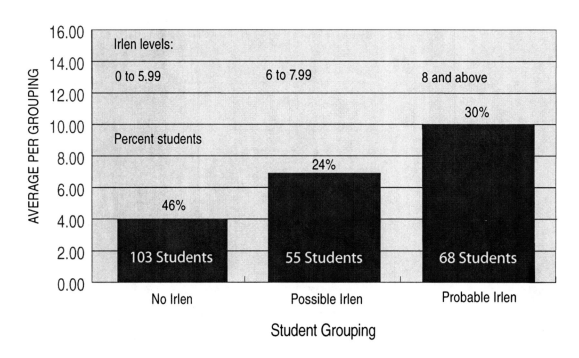

Irlen Assessment—Part A
Data for 226 students

Graph B shows the results from a large, non-random, sample of seven reading, psychology, and sociology classes. Helen Irlen's prescreening instrument for Irlen Syndrome, the "Reading Strategies Questionnaire," was used in this survey. Part A reveals the visual-perceptual dyslexia symptoms that can be caused by Irlen Syndrome.

Graph B

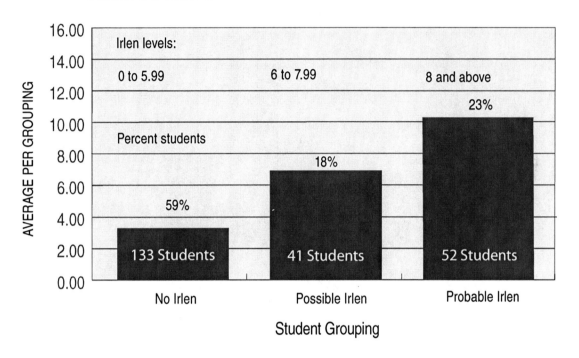

Irlen Assessment—Part B
Data for 226 students

Part B reveals the physical symptoms that can be caused by Irlen Syndrome. Part A indicates that 54 percent of this student sample have visual-perceptual dyslexia symptoms and would benefit from further screening for Irlen Syndrome and / or other types of dyslexia. Part B indicates that 41 percent of this student sample experience physical discomfort when reading and would benefit from additional screening.

Graph C

Student learning modes

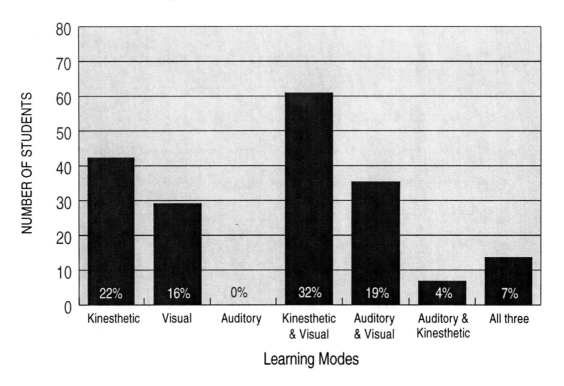

Graph C shows the results from a learning modes survey of 192 psychology and sociology students. Students were asked to indicate their favorite ways to learn: Kinesthetic, Visual, or Auditory. Forty-two students chose the Kinesthetic Modality; 30 students chose Visual Modality; note that only one student of the 192 chose Auditory Modality only. Many students—61—chose both Kinesthetic and Visual Modality; 36 students chose both Auditory and Visual Modality; only seven students chose Auditory and Kinesthetic Modality. Fourteen students indicated that they could learn equally well with any of the three modalities. It is especially significant that only one student of the 192 declared that their favorite way to learn was through lecture only (i.e., Auditory Modality only). More informal surveys conducted over several years with hundreds of students produced similar results.

CHAPTER TWO

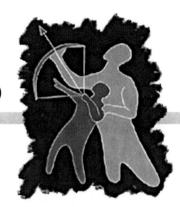

Assessment

How to identify the hidden barriers to reading and learning

My decades of experience as a teacher working with frustrated students have taught me that all students can improve their ability to read, remember, focus, and learn. For many years, I have helped hundreds of discouraged students—ages 10 to 60—overcome handicaps they didn't even know they had. Some students were poor readers because of faulty visual-perceptual brain processing, called "Scotopic Sensitivity Syndrome" or, more commonly now, "Irlen Syndrome." These students have difficulties because their retinas' receptor fields and the visual pathways from their retinas to their brains' visual centers are not "wired" to work well in artificial light and with high-contrast reading materials (Chase, 2005; Irvine, 2005). When these students try to read, their eyes have trouble following along the printed lines, and they may easily lose their place and develop headaches and / or stomachaches. In short, they easily become fatigued when reading.

Other students' auditory pathways cause them to have difficulty connecting the simple sounds they hear with the letter symbols they see when trying to read. Still other students from non-English speaking homes, or homes where reading is not emphasized, experience reading and learning problems when they enter elementary school. If these problems are not addressed, and too often they are not, then these students continue to struggle, become discouraged, and may drop out before completing high school. Students with any—or all—of these problems often are labeled "dyslexic." The prefix "dys" comes from Latin and means "difficult," and the stem word "lexia" comes from Greek and means "words." Together, "difficult words" means that a dyslexic student has trouble reading words (Shaywitz, 2003). Because reading is the cornerstone for all "school smarts," students with any of these problems need the help this book's Basic Program can give them. Students certainly are not helped by the negative labels many have received and, unfortunately, many have not been helped by "special education" programs (Catone & Brady, 2005).

There are also many students who, because of their brain "wiring," have problems paying attention, staying on task, following directions, or remembering. These students often are labeled as having "attention deficit disorder"—or they are labeled as just plain lazy. Evidence from the latest brain research now suggests that these students, too, can benefit from this *Guide*'s free online assessments and suggested remediation exercises that have been shown to "rewire" brains with attention deficits. Cognitive neuroscientists are asking the question, "Can children's brains be trained with computer exercises to improve their ability to pay attention and develop better focusing abilities?" Evidence is now accumulating that answers "yes" to this question. For instance, the eminent cognitive psychologist Dr. Michael Posner has conducted studies on improving the attention abilities of very young children using computer games. Dr. Posner (2003) has stated that "We should think of this work [on attention] not just as remediation but as a normal part of education. Attention plays a very important role in acquisition of high-level skills, and if attention is trainable, it becomes attractive for preschool preparation" (Murray, 2003, p. 58) (Nelson, 1999; Posner & Rothbart, 2005; Vastag, 2007).

Parents should note, however, that their children with visual- or auditory-processing problems, or with inadequate vocabularies, also may have problems paying attention and following directions because they frequently will not be able to understand what they are seeing or hearing. "Attention deficits" then, can have several different causes, and it is important for parents to access *A Practical Guide*'s free Internet assessments and thereby more accurately identify the specific causes for their child's lack of attention and follow-through.

When teachers or schools label students as "disordered," "disabled," or "stupid," they set them up for failure. These labels predict failure and usually cause students great anxiety and shame in learning situations. The result of this labeling, then, *is* failure as students live down to low expectations. Students experiencing difficulty learning to read will begin to think of themselves as unintelligent and will try to hide their difficulty from their peers and parents.

Parents should keep in mind that all students with reading and learning difficulties have the ability to improve their learning if they are assisted with the right programs of instruction and their invisible barriers to learning are identified and remedied (Shaywitz, 2003; Sternberg & Grigorenko, 1999). Recent research reported by Yale University dyslexia specialist Dr. Sally Shaywitz indicates that dyslexic children placed in "a yearlong experimental reading program" experienced remarkable changes in their brain activation patterns and in their reading ability. Dr. Shaywitz (2003) characterizes these changes as "brain repair" (Shaywitz, 2003, pp. 85-86). Furthermore, brain scans of individuals with visual-perceptual dyslexia (Irlen Syndrome) show remarkable improvement when appropriately-colored transparencies are used (Dobrin, 2005; Irvine, 2005).

Unfortunately, many educators still do not know how to recognize and identify specifically these critically important learning barriers. Even more unfortunately, most educators are, often unconsciously, mired in the IQ model. If students don't succeed, even if an invisible handicap like dyslexia is identified and made "visible," many educators believe that such students will always function academically at low levels (Begley, 1996; Martinez, 2000; Neisser, 1998).

In this chapter, I will provide parents with information about how to identify their child's specific reading and learning problems by accessing free Internet website assessments that would cost them hundreds of dollars if they had to hire specialists to assess their child's difficulties. Moreover, very few specialists understand all of the various reading and learning problems that this book will address. Years of research and classroom experience with students have helped me uncover the five central barriers that impede students' reading and learning, and hinder students' academic and eventual workplace success. Many students have more than one of these invisible barriers. These hidden learning barriers are the following, and I will address each in turn:

1) Test anxiety;

2) Visual-perceptual and/or auditory-processing dyslexias;

3) Problems with focus, attention, and staying on task;

4) Working (short-term) memory problems; and

5) Limited or inadequate vocabulary skills.

If parents identify their children's specific learning problems as listed above by using this chapter's free Internet assessments, they will have the information needed to release their children's full learning potential. Furthermore, parents need to remember that IQ tests do not tell the whole story about intelligence and learning abilities. Many students with invisible barriers to learning do not test well. However, by identifying and then removing or diminishing their children's learning barriers, parents will discover and unleash their children's many thinking and learning strengths. In fact, learning specialists like Dr. Sally Shaywitz and Professor Robert Sternberg emphasize the creative and abstract thinking abilities of dyslexic or ADHD students (Davis, 1994; Shaywitz, 2003; Sternberg, 1996).

Assessing students' test anxiety

"Test anxiety alone defeats many of my most dedicated students," I said to my fellow instructors one day at lunch. "I disagree," replied a science teacher, "students just haven't studied, and they use test anxiety as an excuse." This teacher was voicing a belief I have heard often, and one that is commonly voiced by teachers.

However, as a psychologist I am quite familiar with what happens in the brain's memory and learning centers when a person feels anxious—for whatever reason. The body goes into overdrive releasing "fight or flight" hormones. These hormones may have the unwanted effect of wiping out the knowledge the student needs to pass the test. Then, as time ticks away and the class period comes to an end, the student sighs and turns in the test uncompleted. As the student leaves the classroom, hormonal levels are dropping and the test answers begin popping back into the student's mind. This well-researched phenomenon explains why students often protest that they knew the answers but somehow could not retrieve them until too late, i.e., only when the test period was ending (Andreano & Cahill, 2006; Lee, 1999; Sapolsky, 2005, 2000; Shors, 2006).

I tried to explain this physical response brought about by high test anxiety, most often in students who are highly motivated to succeed. "Haven't you had students tell you," I asked the science teacher, "that the test material would suddenly come to mind as they were leaving the classroom?" "Yes," my colleague replied, "I hear this all the time, but I don't believe that these students have some kind of anxiety disease. They just haven't studied well enough." Another colleague, this one a woman math instructor, came to my defense by noting that it was her most motivated female students, particularly in her math courses, who suffered from anxiety's memory-blocking effects. Agreeing with this colleague, I added, "Anxiety's memory-erasing effect is a well-researched phenomenon." Unfortunately, the science teacher remained unconvinced.

I knew that I had failed to remove my science colleague's doubt that many students do study, yet still fail precisely because of high test anxiety. In retrospect, I should have mentioned the research of the distinguished psychologist, Professor Charles Spielberger, who developed anxiety questionnaires that identify students' degree of test anxiety (Spielberger & Associates, 1977). Moreover, Prof. Spielberger researched ways to relieve test anxiety. I also should have reminded my colleagues that many colleges and universities have test-anxiety websites where students can answer a questionnaire to learn about their degree of test anxiety and, in addition, access information about how to overcome it.

If parents believe that high test anxiety is a significant factor preventing their children from doing their best, I recommend that they visit with their child the test-anxiety website of Walla Walla Community College by typing in the Internet address www. wwcc.edu/student_services/online_adv/success/test_test.cfm on their Internet search engine. These key terms should take parents to Walla Walla Community College's online student services website questionnaire and provide them with knowledge about their child's degree of test anxiety. Other college and university websites provide useful suggestions for helping students overcome their test anxiety problems. Survey research I conducted at my Washington State college suggests that nearly half of my college's students have some degree of test anxiety that may be preventing them from working up to their full potential.

My experience, however, is that most students who suffer from high test anxiety have unidentified "invisible" barriers to learning that are the true cause of their anxiety. I have found that removing these hidden barriers also greatly diminishes students' test anxiety. Actually, a little bit of adrenal hormones will help keep students mentally alert (Cahill, & McGaugh, 1998). On the other hand, if students are feeling extremely anxious, then too many stress hormones may be released, and this excessive stress hormone release may block memory retrieval, even when material has been thoroughly memorized (Sapolsky, 2005).

The remainder of this book is devoted to helping parents discover and remove—or at least minimize—their children's specific learning problems. Therefore, the first step for parents is to assess their children by means of the free Internet assessments presented in this chapter and summarized at chapter's end. The second step for parents is to alleviate their children's learning difficulties by means of the remediation exercises suggested in Chapter Three and summarized at the end of that chapter. Finally, parents and their children should revisit the Walla Walla Community College test-anxiety website. After assessment and remediation of the identified learning problems, I am sure that parents will find more confident test-taking children have emerged!

> *For parents who are impatient to get started with the identification and remediation of their child's reading and learning difficulties, I also have provided a very brief overview summary of the Basic Program's assessment and remediation steps with suggestions regarding implementation of the Basic Program at the end of Chapter One, pages 34-36.*

To continue with the identification of specific stumbling blocks, parents next need to gain some understanding about how visual-perceptual and auditory-processing pathways from their children's eyes and ears to areas in their brains may be keeping children from reading and learning to their full academic potential. Genetic malfunctions in sensory and brain systems can give children symptoms of dyslexia and may cause fatigue and even severe headaches when they read (Robinson, 1997; Robinson et al., 2004; Wu, Anderson & Castiello, 2002).

Assessing students' visual-perceptual and auditory-processing problems

For at least 100 years, the term "dyslexia" has been used to refer to children's problems learning to read. More simply, dyslexia has meant an inability to learn to read. In her book, *Overcoming Dyslexia: A New and Complete Science-Based Program for Reading Problems at Any Level*, Dr. Sally Shaywitz (2003) relates how British physicians discovered children who appeared intelligent and eager to learn but who, for unknown reasons, could not learn to read. They used the term "word blindness" to characterize these children's learning problems. During recent decades, learning specialists and brain researchers have found that dyslexia can be caused by many different factors. Dyslexia, however, is not caused by vision problems that require reading glasses. Dyslexia can be caused by problems in the way that the brain processes information, and these problems truly can be invisible—invisible to parents, to teachers, and to the students themselves (Bell et al., 2003; Hamilton & Glasco, 2006; Hudson et al., 2007; McCrory et al., 2005; Shaywitz et al., 2006).

Experts do disagree on the types of dyslexia, as well as on dyslexia's various causes. There is agreement, however, that most problems students experience when learning to read are caused by problems with processing the basic sounds of words. English has 44 basic sounds—or phonemes—which are the auditory building blocks of words. A student's phonemic weakness, most experts agree, is usually genetic in origin (Shaywitz, 2003; Spafford & Grosser, 2005). Some theorists speculate that dyslexics who exhibit this phonemic weakness have brain pathways, called "magnocellular" pathways, which do not process sounds rapidly enough in the brain's hearing pathways. Therefore, these students cannot detect speech sounds spoken rapidly, especially the sounds at the beginnings of words. These students struggle to connect the sounds of words with the letter symbols in words that represent these sounds. Despite this genetic weakness, these dyslexic students are of normal or above-normal intelligence, and many of these students have outstanding strengths in creative and practical intelligence (Chase, 2005; Demonet et al., 2004; Sternberg, 2001).

These slower-than-normal magnocellular pathways are also found in the pathways from the eyes' retinas to the brain's visual cortex. Some researchers now believe that a common type of dyslexia, Irlen Syndrome, is caused by a kind of "visual static" when students with slow magnocellular pathways try to read (Chase, 2005; Harvard Medical School, 1994). Other researchers believe that magnocellular pathways may cause dyslexia because they are involved in the coordination, or working together, of the two eyes (Solan et al., 2003). Magnocellular pathways are also present in the brain's cerebellum, which is responsible for balance, coordination, and some abstract processing. If these pathways malfunction, they may adversely affect visual processing, as well as cause other co-ordination problems responsible for dyspraxia, or the "clumsy child" syndrome (Livingstone et al., 1991; Stordy & Nicholl, 2000).

Still other researchers are investigating the relative size of dyslexics' two cerebral hemispheres and finding that dyslexics have greater hemispheric symmetry than normal readers. By examining brain scans when dyslexics are reading, these investigators also have found that dyslexics rely more on the right hemisphere than normal readers. Normal readers rely on centers in the language-specialized left hemisphere for recognizing sounds, letters, and words. When dyslexic readers try to use their non-language-specialized right hemisphere to read, they have difficulty achieving the automatic word recognition skills that permit reading fluency (Shaywitz, 2003). Finally, the U.S. Navy will soon be releasing the results of their research into visual-perceptual processing that involves the eyes' receptor fields. The Navy's research findings validate the existence of Irlen Syndrome visual-perceptual dyslexia and affirm that 26 percent of the human population has visual receptors (cones) that cannot function well under certain lighting conditions, especially under very bright light or under fluorescent lighting (Irvine, 2005; Parker, 2004).

Although several theories about the primary causes of dyslexia exist, these theories do not necessarily contradict each other because there are several types—and degrees of severity—of dyslexia. It is quite possible that a given student's dyslexia has several causal factors. Many experts think that dyslexics' main difficulty lies in connecting the sounds (phonemes) that they hear to the letters that they see (graphemes). Certainly, the U.S. Navy's research reveals that a major cause of Irlen Syndrome dyslexia lies in the eyes' receptor fields. To further complicate diagnosis, dyslexia may coexist with other hidden barriers to learning, for example, problems with attention. Other reasons for children's lack of reading ability are mentioned by experts who argue that students with reading difficulties may have normal brain "wiring," but may be learning English as a second language, or may have come from families that did not emphasize reading before the child entered kindergarten. Infants and toddlers who are not read to may have impoverished vocabularies and experience greater difficulty learning to read (Chevausky, 1997; Demonet et al., 2004; Gang & Siegel, 2002; Irvine, 2005; Nagarajian et al., 1999; Sternberg & Grigorenko, 1999).

In addition, because reading and learning utilize many brain systems widely dispersed within the brain, interpreting brain scans of a brain-at-work reading or performing other tasks can be problematic. Some experts point to the discovery that some adults who have not learned to read will have brains that, when scanned with new technologies, appear wired like the brains of young dyslexic students. These adults' brains, however, may appear normally wired once they have been taught to read (Sternberg & Grigorenko, 1999). Because of these recent research findings, many reading and learning experts are hesitant to interpret brain scans as able to provide definitive evidence for the causes of dyslexia. Much more research, they argue, is still required to sort out the many confounding variables and conflicting theories about dyslexia's causes—and about the various types of dyslexia.

Parents should keep in mind that visual-perceptual (Irlen Syndrome) dyslexia, ADHD, memory and other cognitive-processing problems are not categorically present or categorically absent. All of these learning problems exist on a continuum and may be present to a mild or to a severe degree. Even if their children are only mildly affected by one of these problems, parents should know that identifying and remediating their child's problem as early as possible can prevent more serious learning difficulties as their child enters higher education.

My own research and experience with students provide me with evidence for at least four causes for dyslexia—all of which can be helped with *A Practical Guide*'s remediation exercises.

- First, dyslexia can be caused by problems in visual-perceptual processing, now usually called Irlen Syndrome.
- Second, dyslexia can be caused by problems in auditory processing, or phonemic weakness.

- Third, dyslexia, or difficulties learning to read, can be caused by English-as-a-second language problems.

- Fourth, lack of reading experiences in infancy and early childhood can handicap a child who is beginning to read.

Irlen Syndrome (IS) and visual-perceptual problems

I have discovered that one of students' most common reading problems involves light-based sensitivities and perceptual distortions. I discovered that many students are especially sensitive to fluorescent lighting and experience difficulty when reading high-contrast materials. This light sensitivity has been investigated in depth by school psychologist and learning specialist Helen Irlen. Irlen Syndrome typically causes dyslexia symptoms in students when they try to read high-contrast material under artificial lighting, and Irlen Syndrome frequently causes physical discomfort and fatigue when reading as well (Irlen, 1994, 2005; Robinson, 1994; Robinson & Foreman, 1999; Stone, 2002).

As I am typing this book on my computer, I have a blue-colored transparency over my computer's screen. This transparency mutes the glare and high contrast of black letters on a white background, thereby permitting me to work longer without fatigue and helping my eyes track more smoothly across the lines and down the page. I am moderately affected by Irlen Syndrome and, therefore, a bit dyslexic. My brain's encoding and decoding of information transmitted by my eyes is such that, without the colored overlay, or my tinted lenses, I would lose my place easily, soon become fatigued, and be unable to continue reading without enormous effort.

Besides fatigue, other physical symptoms of Irlen Syndrome are hurting, red, or itchy eyes; headaches or stomachaches when reading; and / or frequent blinking and squinting. Besides losing one's place, other dyslexia symptoms of Irlen Syndrome are misreading or skipping of words, slow reading speed and problems remembering or comprehending the text. Words appear to shift, or blur, and they appear to move around on the page. Danny, who is more affected by Irlen Syndrome than I am, told

Nan and me after his meeting with Irlen screeners that he saw colored "halos" around each letter. "Why didn't you ever tell us that!" we exclaimed. "I didn't know that other people don't see colored halos around letters," he replied, "until I was questioned during my Irlen screening."

This example should provide parents with insight into why many reading and learning barriers are called "invisible." Everyone assumes that everyone else "sees" or "perceives" the same way they do. Persons with these invisible handicaps have been busy all of their lives compensating by putting forth enormous energy—energy that could have gone into their learning. Unfortunately, for many students seriously affected by Irlen Syndrome, the effort is too much; they simply give up and, often, they drop out of school.

Helen Irlen discovered that students who were having many problems reading in artificial light or with high-contrast materials (black letters on white paper) could read more fluently and with less effort when transparent colored overlays were provided. Starting with blue or red transparent plastic sheets over students' reading materials, Helen Irlen soon developed a method that included a wide range of colors for overlays and for tinted lenses. Her book *Reading by the Colors* tells of her discoveries and of her efforts to eliminate the symptoms that students with Irlen Syndrome were experiencing. Helen Irlen has never claimed that her "colors" method will solve all dyslexia problems, but she does correctly assert that she has found "one piece of the puzzle" (Irlen, 2005). My work with students and my learning differences research have convinced me that providing the right colored overlay for students suffering from Irlen Syndrome constitutes a very *big* piece of the dyslexia puzzle.

Numerous students over the years have reported dramatic improvements in their ability to read, or to stay on task reading difficult texts, when provided with the appropriately-colored overlay. For the young 18-year-old Job Corps student mentioned earlier, as for many others among my students, when the right color is found by the Irlen screener, the results can appear almost miraculous. Indeed, for one middle-aged student, injured at work and returning to school to learn a new trade, the Irlen intervention of appropriately-tinted lenses was life-changing. "If I had known what my learning problem was," he told me, "I would have continued with my education instead of going into construction." This student had been struggling with his mathematics courses. After obtaining his Irlen lenses, he reported that he consistently earned "Bs" in math.

I discovered that another student, diagnosed by psychiatrists with dyslexia and ADD, also had Irlen Syndrome. When she began to use colored transparencies over her computer screen, she reported that the migraines usually accompanying her computer work were gone. Still another student with Irlen Syndrome, aspiring to a degree in nursing, reported that she would become extremely tired and fall asleep only minutes into her nursing textbook. No, she was not bored; she loved her subject, but reading put her to sleep. When she received her colored transparency, however, she told me that she lost track of the time: When she looked up at the clock, she couldn't believe that she had been reading for over two hours without fatigue or drowsiness.

Many students sent to me for evaluation were unaware of the source of their reading problems. Occasionally they would deny having light sensitivity, or tell me that they never thought about it. These are the students who keep visored hats on in the classroom or wear sunglasses indoors. One such student answered my question, "Are you sensitive to light?" with the response, "I don't think so." But when she filled out Helen Irlen's "Reading Strategies Questionnaire," she checked off almost all the boxes marked "frequently," thereby signaling a severe degree of Irlen Syndrome. When the right color overlay was placed on a high contrast printed page, she exclaimed, "Oh, my God! I can see and read this material so much better!" To my amusement, students usually turn to me and ask, "Doesn't that look clearer to you, too?" However, the color that may be the best for one of my students may not be good for me since each individual's color requirement is unique.

Again, most of the hidden barriers addressed by this *Guide* can range from slight to severe. Even when the barrier is not severe, though, students are using brain power and energy to compensate for their problem. This energy would better serve students if used for learning.

What exactly causes Irlen Syndrome?

Harvard Medical School researchers, among others, have uncovered one possible cause of dyslexia symptoms related to Irlen Syndrome in the wiring of the brain's magnocellular visual pathways. There are two visual pathways from the eyes' retinas to the brain's visual cortex. One pathway, the magnocellular, is responsible for high contrast, black and white processing, and is supposed to work rapidly; the other pathway is slower and responsible for processing color. These Harvard researchers found that in some individuals the high-contrast pathway system does not work rapidly enough and may cause something akin to visual "static" or an after-image that interferes with visual processing (Harvard Medical School, 1994).

Although Helen Irlen believes that only about 10-12 percent of individuals have this syndrome, recent research that I and others have carried out with students of various ages in my area of Washington State indicates that a much higher percentage of local students may be affected. For example, I screened 226 college students using Helen Irlen's "Reading Strategies Questionnaire" and found that over 40 percent of them had some degree of Irlen Syndrome (see Graph B, pages 40-41). A controlled study of third-graders in two elementary schools in my area produced similar results, with at least 27 percent of the students having some degree of Irlen Syndrome (students who also may have had Irlen Syndrome but were reading below grade 1.5 were not included in this study). One elementary school's third-graders received their overlays immediately. The other school constituted a control group and received their colored overlays only after three months and they, too, used the overlays for three months (Nobel et al., 2004).

The researchers conducting this study found that the colored overlays brought third-graders above grade level by the end of three months. The students who first received the overlays gained, on average, "grade equivalence scores of between 1 year, 2 months and 1 year, 7 months," while the students who received the overlays three months later "had substantial gains . . . [that] ranged from 1 year, 8 months to 2 years, 8 months," over their three months using the overlays (Noble et al., 2004, pp. 19-20). Students in the second school who were not provided with overlays during the first three months of the study did not make appreciable gains in reading and actually lost nearly half a year in comprehension during that period.

The United States Navy Air Warfare Center's Dr. James H. Irvine has carried out extensive research on the human eye and has reported that Irlen Syndrome is real and that at least 22 percent of the human population is affected by this syndrome. Additional individuals will also exhibit symptoms of Irlen Syndrome under certain lighting conditions. Dr. Irvine's general findings show that "the Irlen effect is real," and that "the energy spectrum presented to the eye of a dyslexic is capable of altering his visual and cognitive performance to a significant extent" (Irlen & Robinson, 1996; Irvine, 2005; Krouse & Irvine, 2003).

Parents can assess whether their children will benefit from the Irlen Syndrome colored overlay intervention, or tinted lenses, by going to Helen Irlen's website, www.irlen.com, for a free assessment and information about obtaining the colored overlays and / or lenses. Hundreds of thousands of individuals, from elementary school age to retirement age, have been freed from crippling headaches and frustrating learning failure by Irlen's colored overlays and tinted lenses. This very important "piece of the dyslexia puzzle," too often an invisible piece, is now becoming more widely recognized as one highly prevalent, but easily remediable, cause of dyslexia symptoms. Helen Irlen has never claimed to "cure" dyslexia, but the Irlen Method does alleviate many troublesome symptoms that prevent students suffering from Irlen Syndrome from wanting to read and, in severe cases, from being able to easily perceive words on the printed page without colored overlays or tinted lenses.

However, there are many brain-based causes of children's dyslexia symptoms that parents can learn about remediating through software exercises specifically designed to lessen these symptoms. For a brief overview of assessments and remediations, parents can consult the summary at the end of Chapter One, pages 34-36, and for more detailed assessment information, they can consult the end of this chapter.

Much still remains for cognitive neuroscientists and learning specialists to learn about the various types of cognitive-processing problems with which students struggle. My own research and work with struggling students have taught me that, like Danny, most students have more than one "genetic glitch" and, in fact, that most learning problems are caused by many genes interacting with many environmental influences. Neuroscientist researchers are finding that there can be more than one cause for many of the symptoms that accompany students' difficulties with reading. For example, students can have problems with decoding and encoding written or spoken words, problems with memory and attention, and problems with words appearing blurred or moving about on the page.

Although for purposes of simplification I have categorized dyslexia as involving visual-perceptual problems or auditory-processing problems, students' brains rely on complex neural networks involving several senses. Students do not learn to read only with their ears or with their eyes; ears and eyes must work together in coordination with the muscle memories from all their body's sensory systems. In fact, the more that brain scientists and learning specialists have increased their knowledge about how the brain reads and learns, the more they have learned about the interdependence of all sensory systems. As one reading specialist has stated, "Teaching reading *is* rocket science" (Louisa Moats quoted in Shaywitz, 2003, p. 258).

Furthermore, the brain develops complex networks in response to environmental stimulation. Ideally, these networks integrate sensory systems and sensory inputs. Unfortunately, for reasons not yet fully understood, not all children have fully coordinated sensory systems: Some systems may malfunction by being under- or over-responsive, or by being connected to each other in unexpected ways. These brain system differences can produce a child with sensory integration problems or with unusual perceptions and creativity (Hartnett et al., 2004; Kranowitz, 2005; Simonton, 2000; Winner, 2000).

Dyslexia categories will undoubtedly change, and many causal hypotheses will be proven incorrect. But success in remediating students' learning and reading difficulties is what counts in the final analysis. After all, aspirin was used to relieve pain for decades before researchers discovered the precise mechanisms through which aspirin worked.

Therefore, my classifying dyslexias as visual-perceptual (Irlen Syndrome) and auditory-processing (primarily phonological difficulties) admittedly represents a simplification of categories. Certainly, reading and learning require the coordination of both visual and auditory systems, as well as many overlapping neural networks in the brain. There is clear evidence that, in many cases of dyslexia, certain pathways existing in several regions of the brain—namely, magnocellular pathways—are malfunctioning (Chase, 2005; Livingstone et al., 1991). The brain sciences will eventually identify and categorize more precisely the various problems students have. For now, parents simply want their children to have help in overcoming their learning problems. Solutions to reading and learning problems are urgently needed now because children are failing when they could be succeeding. *A Practical Guide*'s Basic Program presents effective ways to identify some of the most common reading and learning problems and, above all, effective ways to alleviate many of these common problems.

Auditory-processing problems and dyslexia

Yale University researcher Sally Shaywitz has identified brain areas involved in learning to read. According to Dr. Shaywitz, efficient readers use three areas in the brain's left hemisphere. Dr. Shaywitz's work with brain imaging has revealed that two areas toward the back of the left hemisphere are under-activated in struggling adult readers with dyslexia. Brain imaging of children as young as seven has revealed that this brain under-activity when reading is present in early childhood. Laboratory brain scans of dyslexic adults show the same under-activity patterns as those of younger persons and indicate that this under-activity will not be outgrown—at least not without targeted interventions (Shaywitz, 2003).

Some children read softly aloud to themselves, compensating in this way by activating the brain's language production areas. Others more severely affected may not learn to compensate at all. In addition, the brains of dyslexic children and adults also show greater activity on their brain's right side as their brains are compensating. Shaywitz has found that persons with these brain-based reading problems do not have exact neural models of words built into their brains that allow for automatic word recognition and the reading fluency that this automaticity supports.

Dr. Shaywitz, along with other neuroscientists, emphasizes the "plasticity" of the brain at all stages of life. This means that brains can change and develop, primarily by strengthening communication among nerve cells, and possibly by creating new nerve cells in the brain's learning and memory centers. Therefore, Dr. Shaywitz holds out hope that, even in adults, brain systems that are not functioning efficiently can be improved. She states that although it is better to correct neural systems for reading as early as possible, it is possible to improve the reading fluency and comprehension of adult dyslexics. Dr. Shaywitz stresses that the basic skill required for "exact neural models" of words and for reading fluency and comprehension involves the relationship between the sound of letters—phonemic awareness—and the sight of letter symbols (Shaywitz, 2003).

Not all dyslexia researchers are in complete agreement as to the causes of auditory dyslexia nor do they agree on the remedies required. Irlen Syndrome dyslexia, working memory and attention problems have all been implicated as possible contributing factors (Howes, 2003; Kibby et al., 2004). In addition, the "phonological deficit theory," a dominant theory in auditory dyslexia has produced inconsistent and contradictory findings (Heiervany & Hugdahl, 2003; Johnston & Morrison, 2007; Price & Devlin, 2003). Some researchers, like Rutgers University neuroscientist Paula Tallal, have focused on dyslexic's inability to detect sounds and words auditorily that most individuals can hear. Dr. Tallal's important research into "stretching" speech, that is, slowing down the delivery of sounds and words and then gradually speeding them up (as students' brains are rewired to detect them at normal delivery speeds) has inspired the founding of Scientific Learning's Fast ForWord reading programs. These programs are presently available only to schools and through professionals (Tallal, 1993; Tallal & Benasich, 2002; Tallal et al., 1996; Temple et al., 2000; Travis, 1996).

Therefore, for severely affected dyslexics, I highly recommend Dr. Shaywitz's book, which provides a comprehensive overview of some of dyslexia's causes and the ways that teachers and parents can help dyslexic students. However, I also highly recommend that, as a first step, Irlen Syndrome be eliminated as a possible causal factor for dyslexia symptoms. Dr. Shaywitz discusses several reading programs that are evidence-based, i.e., these programs have proven effective in experimental studies. If children have severe reading difficulties due to dyslexia, then parents may need to investigate the programs presented by Dr. Shaywitz. However, if children are only mildly to moderately affected by dyslexia, then the assessments and remediations suggested by this book may provide the desired reading and learning proficiency.

Parents next need to consider the importance of their children's ability to focus, pay attention, and stay on task while reading and learning.

Assessing students' problems paying attention and completing work

Instructors at all levels of American educational systems have noted an apparent increase in students who have difficulties paying attention in class. There are many theories as to why the number of students with attention deficits has increased; too much television and video-game playing are among the most frequently mentioned causes. Some research from the American Academy of Pediatrics indicates that television viewing increases attention deficits by rewiring infants' and toddlers' brains: The more television children have watched growing up, these researchers claim, the greater are the chances that as students they will have problems paying attention in class (Christakis, 2004).

In addition, researchers note that television programs are frequently interrupted by commercials causing what psychologists call "functional fixedness." Functional fixedness means that children's brains are programmed to pay attention for only brief periods of time. And television and children's video games are fast-paced with highly stimulating sounds and sights that condition children to expect—and even require— ever more intense degrees of stimulation to engage their attention. On the other hand, some research indicates that video and computer-game playing may strengthen some abilities in children, for example, the ability to process visual information more quickly (Dingfelder, 2007). In fact, a growing body of research evidence is demonstrating that computer exercises can improve students' memory, attention, and other thinking abilities (Murray, 2003). *A Practical Guide's* Basic Program is based upon these research findings.

Other, less often mentioned reasons for attention deficits involve nutritional deficits. I will address these in the concluding chapter. The American diet is lacking in certain essential nutrients that support brain growth and functioning. Foremost among these nutrients are the omega-3 fatty acids that used to be supplied when growing children were given cod liver oil. The human brain is 60 percent fat and requires omega-3 fatty acids for the transmission of nervous impulses. When children with attention problems were given fish-oil capsules containing the essential omega-3 fatty acids during research studies conducted at Purdue University, their attention problems were alleviated (Bryan et al., 2004; Stevens, 2000; Stevens et al., 1995; Stordy & Nicholl, 2000).

Children's problems with attention may also reflect experiential deficits because parents may not have had the time to read to their children or to engage them in language-enriching activities. It is well known that children from impoverished backgrounds enter school with vocabularies that are also impoverished as compared to their middle-class peers (Evans, 2004; Hirsch, 2003). Too much time spent watching television and playing video games may also account for the Gallup Organization's previously cited finding that the average 14-year-old in 1950 had a vocabulary of 25,000 words, while in 1999, when the study was rerun, 14-year-olds' vocabulary level had decreased to 10,000 words. Some vocabulary and reading specialists believe that students' vocabulary levels have continued to drop over the past decade. A final reason for the apparent increase in attention deficits may stem from this documented dramatic drop in vocabulary: Difficulty in paying attention certainly can result from students not understanding the words they hear or see (Allen & Sethi, 2004; Chall & Jacobs, 2003).

What is Attention Deficit Hyperactivity Disorder (ADHD)?

Note that the clinical term most often used for attention deficits is ADHD. ADD, meaning "Attention Deficit Disorder," is commonly used, while ADHD refers to problems with attention coexisting with hyperactivity. I prefer not to speak of "disorders" because many persons with ADD, like dyslexic persons, do have above-average intelligence and important strengths. My colleagues in the elementary schools who work with children whose attention deficits and hyperactivity are caused by Fetal Alcohol Syndrome (FAS) or Fetal Alcohol Effects (FAE) inform me that even these children have learning strengths. Whereas ADHD and dyslexia have genetic components that involve differences in the usual brain "wiring," FAS and FAE children have suffered alcohol-induced brain damage. FAS children's brains are more seriously affected than FAE children's brains (Kleinfeld & Wescott, 1993).

Unfortunately, there has been an epidemic in America of alcohol and drug abuse; all too often, pregnant women smoke or become chemically dependent on illegal drugs and / or alcohol. Attention deficits in children certainly can result from the brain damage inflicted on developing fetuses by their smoking and chemically-dependent mothers. However, even these fetal alcohol brain-damaged infants who exhibit attention deficits and hyperactivity at birth may still have brains capable of repair with the use of the exercises suggested in Chapter Three. My colleagues who have worked with Fetal Alcohol Syndrome (FAS) and Fetal Alcohol Effects (FAE) middle-school age children have reported that they found reason for hope when having children with these problems work with the computer exercises this book suggests.

Furthermore, many attention problems are related to genetics; individuals with attention deficit disorder (ADD), or attention deficit hyperactivity disorder (ADHD) often have inherited their brain wiring and brain chemistry. They, like many students with attention deficits, can be above average in intelligence with untapped strengths in creativity and "street smarts." One objective of this *Guide* is to show parents how to help these students strengthen their brains' attention systems so they may better access and use their considerable learning strengths. The good news from the cognitive neurosciences emphasizes the importance of environment and details how stimulating and supportive environments, especially early in a developing child's life, can overcome many genetic and prenatal insults to the brain (Bruer, 1999; Hecker et al., 2002; Lubar et al., 1995; Rollins, 2004).

Stanford University neuroendocrinologist Robert Sapolsky has reported on research with genetically-modified mice who have been bred to be superbright "Doogie" mice, named after the child prodigy TV character, Doogie Howser. By enhancing these lab mice's genetics to endow them with great learning and memory capabilities, Prof. Sapolsky says that a point is scored for the power of genetics to change behavior. Another genetic point is scored, Prof. Sapolsky explains, when researchers produced dim-witted mice by knocking out an important gene. If Sapolsky's story had ended there, parents could come away with reinforcement of the depressing idea that "genetics are destiny." Parents would believe, as many people in our society today do believe, that children born with damaged or diminished brains cannot learn, that they are destined by a roll of the genetic dice, or by prenatal insult, to live a much-diminished life.

Prof. Sapolsky, however, does not end his story there. He recounts an even more interesting research experiment with these genetically dim-witted mice who are placed—as adults—in a stimulating environment. In a superior environment, Sapolsky reports that the dim-witted mice begin to demonstrate greatly improved learning and memory abilities. Nurture, Sapolsky concludes, "scores a come-from-behind victory [over nature] in the final seconds" (Sapolsky, 2000, p. 17A). In the recent past children with "minimal brain damage," as ADHD children were once described, or children who were slow to speak or learn to read, would be written off as "stupid" or "retarded," as indeed some of my college students were. Now, there is a growing body of research demonstrating that the human brain retains its capacity to learn and improve at any age—given a supportive and stimulating environment.

Finally, many learning experts find that problems with staying focused and paying attention are among the most common causes preventing students from fulfilling their academic potential. Dr. Russell A. Barkley, writing in his book *ADHD and the nature of self-control* (1997) has observed that individuals with attention deficits have a "time blindness" that makes it difficult—sometimes impossible—for them to organize and manage time and space. Children with attention deficits need people in their lives to provide a "prosthesis environment" and to help them structure their lives and develop productive routines. Guiding structures act, Dr. Barkley suggests, analogously to glasses for persons with visual problems. Dr. Barkley asserts that it is not that ADHD students do not know what to do; the problem is that they are not able to *do* what they *know*. Inhibition of impulse, follow through, and execution of necessary duties, such as consistent studying and completing homework tasks, present problems for ADHD students, according to Dr. Barkley (Barkley, 1997, pp. 335-350). Again, the importance of supportive environments for the success of ADHD and ADD individuals is emphasized.

The relation of attention deficits to other learning problems

Irlen Syndrome problems—already discussed—can cause both dyslexia symptoms and ADHD symptoms. When children's visual-perceptual processes are defective, they will find reading and paying attention very difficult, and they may have problems sitting quietly in school (Heiervany & Hugdahl, 2003). Parents have already learned how to find out if Irlen Syndrome is affecting their child. I should, however, again emphasize that Irlen Syndrome dyslexia and other dyslexias, as well as ADHD do *not* imply diminished intelligence. Although all of these problems present barriers to reading and learning, they do not reflect below-average intelligence. Many of my students with learning "differences" are intelligent and creative individuals who do, however, struggle academically because of these learning differences.

To help these growing numbers of "nontraditional" students, many of whom are non-English speaking as well as ADHD and/or dyslexic, teachers have tried in recent years to recognize the various learning styles of their students. Teachers are striving to use a variety of teaching methods to reach the increasing numbers of students with learning problems, many of whom are not good visual or auditory learners; rather, many learn best kinesthetically, that is, by doing. Students from working-class or impoverished backgrounds are most often *shown* how to do something by parents, rather than *told* how to do something. In our 21st century's technological societies that demand superior critical thinking and abstract reasoning abilities, kinesthetic learners are greatly disadvantaged.

Certainly, efforts on the part of teachers to reach students who learn kinesthetically or visually, rather than verbally and auditorily, are needed. However, the learning-styles approach to teaching is not adequate to help the large numbers of students who learn best kinesthetically or who may have brain-based learning limitations. Furthermore, the more abstract and advanced the knowledge being taught, the more difficult it is for teachers to teach these abstract concepts kinesthetically. Success in a modern high-tech society requires students to think conceptually, to read fluently, and to pay attention and absorb information that is presented visually and, above all, auditorily. The approach made available to parents and their children by this book does not invalidate a learning styles approach to teaching (which is perfectly appropriate in a child's early years), but the Basic Program outlined within it goes beyond learning styles.

As regards learning styles, educational researchers have not found great differences in learning when students are taught in different modalities. What has been found is that while "modality of instruction is important . . . it is equally important for all students—not more or less important depending on students' modality preference" (Willingham, 2005, p. 34). What is most important is the modality that is best for given content, that is, "each modality is effective in carrying certain types of information" (Willingham, 2005, Ibid.). Students learn how to build a birdhouse or play the flute best through the kinesthetic modality of building birdhouses and playing flutes, and not simply by reading "how to" manuals. More abstract concepts of morality and justice—even for younger students—are best learned through stories, lectures, and debate, although classroom analysis of movies and stories, and role-playing can combine several learning modalities to good effect.

A Practical Guide's Basic Program is significant because it shows parents how to expand their children's learning modality repertoire by enlarging the capacity of their children's brains. The Basic Program makes full use of the latest cognitive neuroscience research and presents parents with the means to "rewire" their children's brains with computer exercises (Chenausky, 1997; Horgan, 1996; Murray, 2003; National Institutes of Health, 1998; Posner & Rothbart, 2005; Rossiter & La Vaque, 1995; Sands & Buchholz, 1997; Science News, 2004, 2001; Travis, 1996).

The effective exercises presented in Chapter Three have been shown to improve children's attention, memory, reading, and learning abilities. When children employ the recommended computer software remediation exercises, they can expand the ways in which their brains can access and process information. These children will have multiplied the number of learning-style modalities they possess.

How parents can assess if their child has ADHD or ADD

Attention deficit, like Irlen Syndrome and dyslexia, is a *spectrum* problem; this means that the problem is found on a continuum, ranging from mild through severe. Some students are very mildly affected, some students more moderately, and some students quite severely. In addition, research reveals that when ADHD or ADD is present, about 50 percent of children will harbor other learning difficulties as well (Barkley, 1997).

Because students are affected to different degrees, they "hit their ceiling," i.e., reach the limits of their ability to compensate, at different points in their education. A mildly affected student with only one problem may not feel slowed down until senior high school—or even college. A severely affected student might be struggling already, and failing, in elementary school. One of my creative and articulate college students confided to me that she had been labeled "retarded" in grammar school. With her self-esteem demolished, she dropped out of high school, got married, and had children. Flourishing in the practical world of family and work, she began to realize that she was not stupid. When her gifted son was diagnosed with ADHD and dyslexia, she recognized her own learning differences, and she resolved to find ways for both of them to learn. She returned to school, completed a high school equivalency degree, an AA, and a BA in special education. Her story, like that of so many other students who have struggled to overcome invisible handicaps and negative labels, can inspire parents to identify and diminish their children's academic stumbling blocks before these handicaps and labels damage their children's self-confidence and self-esteem.

Because ADHD is one of the most common problems affecting students today, and because less severe forms of ADD, especially, may not be easily diagnosed, parents would be well advised to visit the website of Dr. Daniel G. Amen, one of the world's most accomplished brain researchers. Dr. Amen has generously provided free online assessments for ADHD and ADD. A highly respected neuropsychiatrist and a specialist in scanning brains with the latest methods, Dr. Amen has found that ADHD comes in several types. Dr. Amen's ADHD subtype assessment will inform parents of the possibility—or probability—that their child has a given ADHD subtype. Once parents have completed Dr. Amen's subtype assessment, they can access the diet, supplements, and medications required to alleviate their child's specific type of ADHD. This information would cost hundreds of dollars if provided by a psychiatrist, and most psychiatrists do not have this information to dispense. Dr. Amen's ADHD subtype information is especially critical information because Dr. Amen has discovered that the diet and supplements helpful for one ADHD subtype may worsen the symptoms for other types (Amen, 1998).

By going to Dr. Amen's website, *www.amenclinic.com*, parents can discover if their child may have some degree of attention deficit. They also can identify the specific ADHD subtype that may be involved. In addition, this website provides parents with the many resources Dr. Amen makes available. Dr. Amen's books, videos, and audiotapes contain indispensable information about better thinking and better learning, even for individuals who do not have ADHD.

Assessing students' working-memory problems

Thus far, I have indicated how parents can assess their children for Irlen Syndrome and access more information about other types of dyslexia. The research I have cited estimates that at least 20 percent—and possibly 26 percent—of humans have the visual-perceptual problems caused by the genetics of Irlen Syndrome. For reasons that yet have to be discovered, as many as 40 percent or more of children growing up in many areas of America may be affected by Irlen Syndrome. Besides genetic factors, poor nutrition, especially a lack of essential fatty acids in children's diets, appear implicated. Dr. Sally Shaywitz estimates that between 20 percent and 30 percent of American children struggle when learning to read and that at least one in five (20 percent) of these children have some degree of auditory-processing dyslexia (Shaywitz, 2003). Many students may be struggling with both visual-perceptual and auditory-processing dyslexia. Magnocellular dysfunction, implicated by some researchers in relation to Irlen Syndrome, could also contribute to auditory-processing dyslexia because magnocells are found in the areas of the brain's primary auditory cortex as well as in the cerebellum (Beatty, 2001).

In his statement to the U.S. Senate's Committee on Labor and Human Resources, "Overview of Reading and Literacy Initiatives," Dr. G. Reid Lyon, Past Director of the Child Development and Behavior Branch within the National Institute of Child Health and Human Development, made the following statement: "Unfortunately, it appears that for about 60% of our nation's children, learning to read is a much more formidable challenge [than for the others], and for at least 20% to 30% of these youngsters, reading is one of the most difficult tasks that they will have to master throughout their schooling" (Lyon, 1998, p. 1). Dr. Lyon emphasizes that, for most children, failure to easily learn to read demonstrates to them, and to their classmates, that they are not intelligent, no matter the reasons—often hidden—for their failure. Parents can now begin to understand how critically important it is to help their children avoid reading failure by identifying as soon as possible the sources of their children's difficulties and removing these difficulties to the greatest extent possible.

Experts disagree on the percentages of American students struggling to overcome ADHD, but most experts would agree that we do live in an "ADDogenic" society, with many factors contributing to an increase in this often invisible learning problem (Hallowell & Ratey, 2006, 1994). Most experts also agree that many individuals who are mild-to-moderately affected by ADD may struggle all of their lives without ever being properly diagnosed. Parents now have at their disposal the means to assess their children for ADHD subtypes.

In addition to the many unidentified students who may be struggling silently with various types of dyslexia and ADHD, and therefore not easily learning to read, my research and teaching experience have shown me that students also struggle with other related cognitive-processing problems, especially problems involving short-term, or working memory. Therefore, before presenting an excellent free Internet site for assessing and remediating memory and attention problems, I want to briefly explain memory types and their important role in learning.

The three kinds of memory

Cognitive psychologists study memory. They research the kinds of memory systems humans have and how memories are processed by the brain. Although there are controversies in memory research and disagreements among memory researchers, there is much agreement as well. Most cognitive psychologists agree that there are three different kinds of memory: First, there is *immediate*, or *sensory, memory* that registers a great amount of detail in the visual, auditory, and touch sensory registers for only a couple of seconds. If a person is motivated to pay attention to some of these sensory details, then the second memory system, *short-term*, or *working, memory* becomes activated.

Working memory can hold limited amounts of information for a few seconds without rehearsal. Most people can hold about seven different pieces of information for longer periods if they are rehearsing or "working" with the information they are holding in working memory. Therefore, working memory has been likened to a computer desktop: Individuals activate a portion of the problem they are working on; they retrieve elements for consideration from the storage areas of memory, the memory system called *long-term memory* and, with "desktop working" of these elements, they solve their problem. Long-term memory, then, is the third kind of memory system and is said to be relatively permanent, with huge, perhaps infinite, storage capabilities.

My research with students has taught me to be particularly concerned about their working-memory capabilities. Studies of working memory have found that some individuals' working memory can only hold five pieces of information—or less—at a time, while other individuals' working memory can hold nine pieces of information at a time. The key factor for problem-solving, reading comprehension, and long-term storage of information is the efficiency of students' working memories. For example, poor auditory or visual working memory translates into problem-solving, comprehension, and retention difficulties. If a student can hold only a few elements in working memory, then incorporating these elements into long-term storage becomes difficult, if not impossible.

Countless students have complained to me that they have such poor auditory memories that by the time lecturers have arrived at the end of their sentences, they have already forgotten what was said at the beginning. For students with such poor auditory working memories, good note taking is impossible. Parents can refer again to Graph C on page 42, where the results of student surveys convey dramatically how very few are the students who can learn easily through lecture only. Graph C formally represents but a small portion of the students I have surveyed in all my classes, year after year, with a more informal show of hands. The results are always the same: Those students who have auditory working memories efficient enough to serve them well in college learning situations are almost nonexistent. My colleagues in the elementary, middle, and high schools report similar findings: Their students, too, have difficulty remembering what they hear.

Cognitive neuroscience research supports what my work with students has taught me, namely, that enlarging the capacity of auditory (and visual) working memory can facilitate reading comprehension, problem-solving, and retention. Retaining and understanding what is learned becomes easier, and comprehension is greatly improved as working memory is improved. Some students have good visual working memory capabilities and poor auditory working memory capabilities; some students struggle with poor working memories in all sensory modalities. The vast majority of my students have poor auditory working memories: They are not good lecture-only learners.

Why do students have problems with working memory?

There are many reasons for the difficulties students have with remembering what they have just heard long enough to move the information into their long-term memory stores. Some of them are cultural. Our American culture is a fast-food, sleep-deprived culture, and today's generations of students are raised on fast-paced, highly stimulating, and rapidly changing television shows, video games, and other entertainment forms. Our students' brains are conditioned to seek high levels of stimulation that are constantly and rapidly changing. Brain studies reveal that these forms of entertainment produce passive brains and engender addiction-like cravings that have taken the place of the concentration and active processing demanded by reading and learning. In addition, a sleep-deprived student's memory will not retain information as well as a rested student's memory. Finally, I stress the importance of supplying students' brains with the proper nutrients, especially the omega-3 fatty acids and B vitamins required for optimal brain functioning. Nutrition research shows that most American students' brains are not receiving the nutrients essential for optimal learning performance, and many American students are lacking in essential minerals like iron, calcium and zinc (Stevens, 2000, 1995; Stordy & Nicholl, 2000).

Moreover, if students have visual-perceptual problems, such as Irlen Syndrome dyslexia, they will have problems with their working memory, focus, and the attention necessary to move information into their long-term memory stores (Wickelgren, 2001). For these students, learning occurs with difficulty or not at all. Students who have inherited some degree of auditory-processing dyslexia and have trouble connecting the phoneme (letter sound) that they hear with the grapheme (letter symbol) that they see will have problems with oral and written language. They will avoid reading and will have weak auditory-processing abilities.

Students who have a genetic tendency towards some degree of attention deficit or who have had attention deficits culturally programmed into their brains (or both!) will have poor working memories. Students who have not become regular readers, for any of these reasons, will have a continuing and worsening struggle to become effective learners, and, as a result, they will have impoverished vocabularies, in addition to their other learning problems. Further, students with poor working memories may experience problems with math performance and anxiety (Ashcraft & Kirk, 2001).

Parents will undoubtedly recognize if their child does have weaknesses in auditory working memory and may even have ideas regarding other cognitive-processing areas that their child needs to strengthen.

For assessing a child's working memory and other cognitive-processes important for academic success, parents will find help through the diagnostic questionnaire designed by Dr. Frederick Weiner, Parrot Software's CEO. Dr. Weiner has been designing remediation and rehabilitation software for memory, attention, reasoning, and communication for over 25 years. Although Dr. Weiner's programs are targeted at rehabilitating older persons with brain injuries, cognitive decline due to Alzheimer's, other dementias, and aging, many educational institutions find his memory and attention programs equally effective for students of all ages. Dr. Weiner has taught speech pathology in major colleges and universities, and his brain-retraining programs have been used by schools and institutions, as well as by individuals throughout the U.S. and Canada, as well as internationally.

Parents can access Dr. Weiner's diagnostic questionnaire for memory, reasoning, word recall, and vocabulary at www.parrotsoftware.com. Dr. Weiner's excellent diagnostic questionnaire is free online. After students have taken this assessment, they are provided with information regarding their specific cognitive-processing weaknesses, as well as Parrot Software's remediation exercises shown to effectively strengthen these deficient areas. The Basic Program that I present in Chapter Three indicates the remediation exercises that I have used and found most effective for helping students strengthen their auditory working memory and attention.

As a former university professor and speech pathologist who has worked for decades helping students and clients overcome their cognitive-processing deficits, Dr. Weiner understands how important self-confidence and self-esteem are to students who have struggled—some, all their lives—with learning problems. Therefore, Dr. Weiner emphasizes that all of his learning programs are easy to understand, and that his remediation exercises, while challenging and effective, are never boring or intimidating. Even very young children, or older adults who have never used a computer, will find themselves stimulated as Parrot Software exercises engage their minds, and as they feel their brains' capabilities improving. I should mention that all of the software recommended in Chapter Three's Basic Program are as inexpensive as they are effective.

Assessing students' vocabulary levels

I cannot emphasize too much that American students need to develop their word power if they wish to achieve academic success and, ultimately, experience success in today's high-tech workplace. Students' word power—the strength and extent of their vocabularies—will determine quite literally how far they can go in school and later in their professions. Over the last 50 years, well-conducted surveys reveal a disturbing drop in the size of young high-school students' average vocabularies. Teachers at all levels report that students are not reading as much as they should to develop their vocabularies. Learning specialists assert that after about the sixth grade, it is only through reading that students increase the size of their vocabularies (Shaywitz, 2003). College instructors across this nation, from those at community colleges to those at elite Ivy League universities, complain that entering students are not prepared for college work or to understand college-level textbooks (Manno & Finn, 1996; Roueche & Roueche, 1999).

When I was a beginning doctoral student at the University of California, Irvine, the lead professor for my interdisciplinary group, Prof. Stanley Aronowitz, stressed that "learning the lingo is 90 percent of the battle in any discipline." I never forgot his words. When I started teaching in my Washington State community college, located in an impoverished, rural part of the state, I immediately became aware of my students' poor vocabularies. True, many of my students were English-as-a-second-language students, mainly Spanish-speaking, with a few foreign students from Japan. However, almost as often, the students struggling with basic vocabulary deficits were dominant-culture students, many from working-class families, and some from middle-class families.

Most of the students did not know why they could not understand their college-level texts; they tended to blame their teachers when they failed to do well on multiple-choice quizzes or essay exam questions. About the time that I began to recognize their lack of college-level vocabularies, the older returning woman student I mentioned earlier came to me after class, asking for help: "Dr. Morrow," she pleaded, "Please tell me what to do. My mother only had a third-grade education, and *I just don't have the words!*" This plump, pleasant-looking, gray-haired woman was obviously desperate for a solution to her educational impasse. I have never forgotten her pleas. This book's Basic Program of assessment and remediation represents the answer I have developed for her and for all of the many struggling students like her of all ages who "just don't have the words."

Why are American students so lacking in vocabulary power?

There are many environmental and genetic brain-based reasons why our American students don't read anymore. And since they don't read, they can't possibly "have the words." In addition, students for whom English is a second language often are illiterate in their native tongue: They can't read either Spanish, for example, or English with speed and accuracy. Some of these students also struggle with the syndromes that I have already mentioned. They may have the visual-perceptual processing problems that signal Irlen Syndrome dyslexia, and, therefore, they find that reading is literally painful for them. In addition, they may have various degrees of auditory-processing dyslexia and/or ADHD that make reading tiresome and difficult.

Furthermore, students from poverty-level or working-class families often are not read to by their parents in early childhood. Parents in these families are struggling to obtain the basic necessities for their children and may be stressed and limited in the time they have to spend reading to their children. Many parents are unaware of the critical importance of reading to, and with, their children so that their children will develop the abilities required for academic success. Typical mother-child interactions in such families are by *showing* rather than by *telling*. When such children enter school, their vocabularies already lag far behind their middle-class and English-speaking peers, and it is difficult for them to ever catch up without the kind of interventions this book presents (Hart & Risley, 2003).

I was naïve to think that the relationship between the socioeconomic levels of students and their vocabulary development was known to all educators, especially to my colleagues in my college's English department. One day, I was speaking about this relationship to one of my most competent colleagues, an instructor of developmental English. I began mentioning the relationship between socioeconomic level and vocabulary, and I stated what I thought was a well-known fact, namely, that working-class mothers tend not to talk much to their children. To my surprise, my colleague exclaimed, "You mean that many of our entering students' vocabulary levels do not permit them to access our college-level texts!" I could see that this idea was a revelation to her. For me, the revelation was that a college English instructor did not realize just how impoverished her students' vocabularies actually were.

Reading experts emphasize that by the end of third grade students must be ready to transition from "learning to read" to the fourth grade's "reading to learn." However, as I have argued, increasing numbers of American students at all levels have visual-perceptual and auditory-processing difficulties, as well as ADD or ADHD, in addition to limited vocabularies that handicap them. These students' invisible barriers to fluent reading and learning cause them to fail or to underachieve in school and, later, on the job. The good news from the cognitive neurosciences is that these invisible barriers now can be made visible; the even better news is that, once visible and identified, these barriers can be removed, or at least greatly minimized.

How to determine students' vocabulary levels

Parents can learn how to identify their child's vocabulary level by visiting the Internet website of WordSmart, a company that has produced effective and fun vocabulary-building software and is, in my opinion, the best vocabulary-building software available. WordSmart's website, www.wordsmart.com, will tell parents about the effective and amusing computer games that children can play to rapidly improve their word knowledge. At the website, www.wordsmartedu.com, parents can experience WordSmart program demos. Both of WordSmart's websites provide parents with a free vocabulary assessment in the form of a game, "Take the WordSmart Challenge." Using this assessment, parents can identify the appropriate WordSmart volume and the word group within that volume at which to most profitably begin their children's vocabulary building.

For preschool through second grade, WordSmart offers an award-winning phonics package. Vocabulary-building packages are also available for grade school (first grade through fifth grade), for middle school (fifth grade through ninth grade), and for high school students (ninth grade through twelfth grade). WordSmart also offers excellent vocabulary-software programs for adults and for English-as-a-second-language learners.

WordSmart is a company that utilizes the Johnson O'Connor Foundation's 70 years of research carried out by testing over a million subjects. Dr. Johnson O'Connor is considered the father of aptitude testing. Harvard-educated, Dr. O'Connor became the head of electrical engineering for the General Electric Company, where he led research into aptitudes and appropriate job placement. O'Connor's research found evidence supporting the link between individuals' vocabulary levels and their academic and workplace success. His foundation's many decades of research developed the vocabulary-learning principles that are the foundation for WordSmart's effective computer software programs.

Once parents have identified the appropriate programs for their children, they can learn more about WordSmart's vocabulary remediation software at the end of Chapter Three.

Summary of the Basic Program for assessment

The following five steps are critical in identifying children's specific invisible barriers to reading and learning success. These steps are the foundation of the Basic Program for assessment. With each step, I provide the appropriate "tool" (i.e., website) to accomplish the respective assessment.

Step 1. Assessing children's test anxiety: Test anxiety defeats many students before they even begin. Test anxiety often masks significant problems in brain-processes that make reading and learning difficult. I've found that removing these brain-processing problems will lessen test anxiety.

Parents can assess their children both before and after applying the Basic Program remediations: Find Walla Walla Community College's test anxiety questionnaire online at http://www.wwcc.edu/student_services/online_adv/success/test_test.cfm.

Step 2. Assessing children for Irlen Syndrome dyslexia (visual-perceptual processing problems): The visual-perceptual processing difficulties caused by Irlen Syndrome can manifest as serious eye strain, headaches, and fatigue while reading high-contrast materials, especially under artificial lighting conditions. Students with Irlen Syndrome often have symptoms of dyslexia, such as misreading, poor comprehension, and frequently losing their place, as well as fatigue when reading. For students with other types of dyslexia, there are emerging remediation technologies that will be addressed in Chapter Three.

Parents can assess their children for Irlen Syndrome at the Irlen International Institute's free Internet website: www.irlen.com.

Step 3. Assessing for attention-deficit problems: Brain-based attention-deficit (ADHD and ADD) problems appear to be increasing among American students. These problems with focus and staying on task are among the most common, usually invisible, barriers to learning. ADHD and ADD can vary from very mild to quite severely handicapping.

Even mild attention deficits can diminish students' ability to work up to their full academic potential.

Parents can assess their children for ADHD and ADD problems at www.amenclinic. com.

Step 4. Assessing for memory difficulties: Short-term or working-memory problems, along with other cognitive-processing problems, affect many students of all ages. My research and experience have taught me that it is a rare student who can claim a "photographic" visual memory or who can hear something once and remember it forever. Learning can take place only when a student's short-term memory works well enough for information to be encoded and stored in long-term memory.

Parents can assess their children's memory and other cognitive processes at www. parrotsoftware.com, where they can experience the free memory and attention-building software demonstrations provided. Parrot Software programs were developed by Dr. Frederick Weiner, a former speech pathologist at Pennsylvania State University, in conjunction with clinical specialists who worked with individuals experiencing memory, attention, and reasoning deficits. Dr. Weiner founded Parrot Software in 1981 and, since that time, has seen his over 60 programs used with great success in many educational and rehabilitation centers throughout the United States, as well as around the world. Dr. Weiner's programs have been translated into five languages. Although Dr. Weiner's website emphasizes "rehabilitation," parents should be reassured that many educational institutions use his programs to remediate students' problems with memory.

Parents can take the "Communication Survey" with their children to find areas that need remediation (also see my remediation program suggestions for memory at the end of Chapter Three and in the appendixes). Parents and children can experience the programs by clicking on "demos."

Step 5. Assessing vocabulary level: An impoverished vocabulary is the inevitable outcome for students harboring problems with their visual- and auditory-processing systems, ability to focus and pay attention, and with their working memory and other cognitive-processing abilities. Reading is difficult and fatiguing for such students, and retaining what they have read is often nearly impossible. Poor vocabularies are also common in students who are English-language learners or who come from families that, for whatever reason, have not emphasized reading.

Parents can learn how to assess their children for vocabulary level at www.wordsmart. com, where they will gain knowledge about how much their children need to grow their vocabularies, and how they can help their children do just that.

By identifying their children's reading and learning barriers, parents will better understand their children and their children's academic struggles. Parents will better understand why their children, depending on the degree of severity of these barriers, may suffer from low self-esteem and why their children may be hesitant at times to tackle new learning. Sadly, students who harbor significant weaknesses in one area often suffer from inadequacies in other areas. These learning difficulties can cause children's low self-esteem and can also be the source of many behavioral problems.

Fortunately, research emerging from the cognitive neurosciences has demonstrated that the human brain is "plastic" at all stages of the lifespan. This means that ways exist to strengthen defective brain connections and that specially-designed computer exercises can rewire the brain to overcome lacks in attention, focus, and working memory. Also available now are computer games and exercises that make rapid vocabulary acquisition easy and fun.

Suggested Reading

For Irlen Syndrome
Besides Helen Irlen's classic text, *Reading by the colors: Overcoming dyslexia and other reading disabilities through the Irlen method* (2005), another excellent source on Irlen Syndrome is:

Stone, R. (2002). *The light barrier: A color solution to your child's light-based reading difficulties.* New York: St. Martin's Press.

For auditory-processing dyslexia
Shaywitz, S., M.D. (2003). *Overcoming dyslexia: A new and complete science-based program for reading problems at any level.* New York: Alfred A. Knopf.

Sternberg, R. J., & Grigorenko E. L. (1999). *Our labeled children: What every parent and teacher needs to know about learning disabilities.* Cambridge, MA: Perseus.

For ADHD and general improvement of the brain
Amen, D. G., M.D. (2005). *Making a good brain great: The Amen Clinic Program for achieving and sustaining optimal mental performance.* New York: Random House.

Hallowell, E.M., M.D., & Ratey, J.J., M.D. (2006).*Delivered from distraction: Getting the most out of life with attention deficit disorder.* New York: Ballantine Books.

Hallowell, E.M., M.D., & Ratey, J.J., M.D. (1994). *Driven to distraction: Recognizing and coping with attention deficit disorder from childhood through adulthood.* New York: Pantheon Books.

Two excellent general sources on learning difficulties and the brain for parents and teachers are
Brubaker, C. L. (2005). *L.D. from the inside out: A survival guide for parents.* Casper, WY: Whiskey Creek Press.

Johnson, L-A. (2005). *Teaching outside the box: How to grab your students by their brains.* San Francisco: Jossey-Bass.

CHAPTER THREE

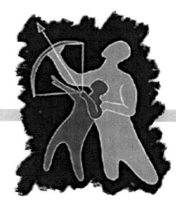

Remediation
How to minimize or eliminate barriers to learning

In Chapter Two, I addressed the problems that test anxiety poses for children, along with how to prevent and eliminate such fear. Students with invisible barriers to reading and learning are often unaware that those problems are slowing them down—despite their best efforts to keep up with their peers. At first pretending not to care that they are falling behind, these students silently suffer from eroding self-esteem and believe that they are just not as smart as their peers. They may eventually give up and become school dropouts with emotional problems that hinder them in every life arena. Those who do stay in school may become "class clowns" with behavioral problems that disrupt learning in their classrooms.

Struggling students frequently suffer from unidentified learning differences which, when added to childhood's normal stresses, may result in high test anxiety, perceived failure, and unfulfilled potential. Children's perceptions of failure soon develop into actual failure in academic achievement and social relationships. At times, parents, in their frustrated efforts to help a bright child who is not achieving academically, will berate and / or punish the child. In these instances, parents think that their punishments and criticism will motivate their child to work harder. As this book makes clear, children with hidden barriers to reading and learning need *encouragement*, not disparagement. I remember a story that one of my dyslexic students told me she had read about an elementary-school-age boy who was struggling with reading. This boy's very critical father took his son to a psychologist who was also a learning specialist. After spending time with the boy, whom the father had accused of lacking motivation, the psychologist presented the father with a page of garbled text. "Read this," the psychologist told the father. "I can't read this!" exclaimed the father, "The words are all jumbled and don't make sense!" "That's how your son sees the page," replied the psychologist. The father suddenly "saw" and understood his son's reading difficulties and broke down in tears. "And I recognized myself in that little boy," was my dyslexic student's quiet conclusion.

Few parents would treat their children as this father had treated his severely dyslexic son, but all parents need to recognize that a child with behavioral problems and struggling in school is all too often a child with unidentified learning problems. If parents can use *A Practical Guide* to identify and diminish or eliminate their children's barriers to reading and learning, then many behavioral problems will also diminish and may even disappear. Children who are successful in their classrooms will generally develop high self-esteem and positive social relationships (O'Neil Bona & Martin, 2004).

Remediation Program

Once parents have identified their children's learning difficulties, they will be ready to embark with them on implementing a specific remediation program. Children who have been struggling for years respond enthusiastically to this *Guide's* brain-building exercises when parents are supportive and communicate their belief in their children's ability to improve their thinking skills. Once children have followed their computer exercise programs for a few hours, they begin to sense their growing capabilities. Children also can follow their progress objectively because progress reports are provided by the software programs. Children—and even adult students!—especially enjoy the "laser review game," which is the last exercise in the WordSmart exercise series. They invariably apply themselves to mastering their vocabulary words so they may enter the "asteroid field" and use the laser to shoot down the asteroids labeled with their words' synonyms.

The Parrot Software exercises are equally engaging and effective. Children playing these games during pilot studies have exclaimed "That's cool!" Before long, children begin to experience in the classroom the gains brought to them by the Basic Program. Students in my pilot studies have gained at least one year of grade level in reading after an hour a day, four days a week for six weeks. Many students have gained four to five grade levels in reading during this period of time. As students begin to recognize the effectiveness of these programs, typically they complete the exercises with a growing recognition of their own competencies and an increasing desire to master their classroom assignments.

Step 1. Remediating students' visual-perceptual problems

I have discovered that Irlen Syndrome is one of the most common unidentified problems afflicting students. Many more students than commonly recognized by specialists are sensitive to artificial light and to high-contrast reading materials. This sensitivity to certain light frequencies constitutes a "light barrier" that can make reading and learning not only difficult, but nearly impossible, depending on the degree to which a given student is affected (Driscoll, 2004; Irlen, 2005; Stone, 2002).

If students are mildly affected by Irlen Syndrome, then an adequate intervention might be for them to avoid reading under artificial lighting. However, most of my students who are light sensitive do better once they begin using the correct colored transparency over their reading materials. Chapter Two encouraged parents to have their children fill out the free Irlen Syndrome self-assessment available on Helen Irlen's Internet website (www.irlen.com). The U.S. and international locations of Helen Irlen's clinics are available on the Irlen website, along with many other reading aids. In addition, by referring to this website, parents can find Irlen's trained screeners who work with Irlen Syndrome-affected individuals to find the most effective color transparency to place over reading materials and computer screens.

When Danny had his screening, I was surprised by the wide range of colors that different individuals may require. I was equally surprised to learn that the color required for tinted lenses, or tinted reading glasses, might vary considerably from the color needed for an overlay. As a serious student, Danny used his eyes constantly for studying and for school-related computer work. Therefore, Nan and I decided to have Danny screened by an Irlen diagnostician for tinted reading glasses. With his Irlen tinted lenses, Danny's academic work improved significantly and his headaches and fatigue when reading disappeared. When I had my own Irlen diagnostic screening, I was surprised to discover that the world did not take on the color of the lenses I found most helpful. When I looked through the lenses with my best color, a blue-grey, the world looked normal to me, and I did not become tired as I usually did when I read for long periods. The fatigue and sleepiness I would experience shortly after starting to read dissipated.

Colleagues who were skeptical about the existence of Irlen Syndrome would have a hard time convincing individuals with Irlen Syndrome about its non-existence because these individuals have experienced, as did Danny, my students, and I, the tremendous benefits of Helen Irlen's interventions.

Whether students obtain lenses tinted in their best color, or just an appropriate overlay for texts and computer screens, they will find that their ability to read without headaches or fatigue—and, best of all—their ability to comprehend and remember what they read will be greatly improved.

A typical example of academic improvement brought about by the Irlen intervention occurred when one of my most capable students came to me complaining about his inability to understand fundamental math concepts. Assessments revealed him to have high intelligence and severe Irlen Syndrome. This student was greatly relieved to be reassured he was intelligent because his hidden learning barriers had filled him with self-doubt about his ability to achieve academic success. He was, in fact, delighted to discover his primary learning problem was severe Irlen Syndrome. During assessment, the Irlen diagnostician found that my students' eyes were following the letters that appeared to him to be bouncing around on the page so much that he was continuously miscopying numbers, just as he misread and misunderstood math problems. Because of the severity of his problem, this student decided to obtain tinted lenses.

When I next encountered him, my student happily told me that "being informed that I was capable and intelligent, along with obtaining Irlen tinted lenses dramatically changed my self-concept and my life." He said that he wished he had known years ago what he now knows about why he had problems reading in both middle and high school. "If I had known that I had Irlen Syndrome, and if I had known how easily this stumbling block to learning could be removed," he said, "my whole life up until this moment would have been very different because I would not have become a construction worker; I would have continued with my education as I am now successfully doing." Finding and correcting this older, returning student's main learning problem raised his low grades to a high "B" level and ensured his college graduation and a future in our high tech society.

Many students with Irlen Syndrome or other types of dyslexia easily lose their place when reading. A striking illustration of this problem came from one of my colleagues. I had been impressed with this colleague's brilliant mind and exceptional teaching abilities and was surprised when he told me that he has both Irlen Syndrome and auditory-processing dyslexia. My colleague confided that he would not have been able to finish high school, let alone go on to higher education for a doctorate, if, as he stated, "a teacher had not given me the finger." This colleague's students are always amused when he tells them how a teacher helped him by "giving me the finger," but behind my colleague's disarming humor, he was making a serious point. The teacher who changed his life gave him the simple reading intervention of following along the printed line with his finger. This one suggestion, along with the teacher's belief in my colleague's ability to succeed, set him on the path to becoming a competent learner.

My colleague is now a professional with a master's degree, and he has completed most of his doctoral studies. He told me that without his teacher's intervention and belief in him, he is certain that he would have become a high school dropout.

The Irlen website contains information about many other aids to reading, including specially designed colored and transparent bars that can be moved along a line of text to help students keep their place. These bars function to remediate students for Irlen Syndrome much like "the finger," but also much more effectively. Hats with visors can be worn when working under fluorescent lights and, of course, colored overlays can be used over printed material or over a computer screen. Some instructors are offended when students wear hats in the classroom. I have discovered, however, that many of these students suffer from light sensitivity and are using hats with visors to shade their eyes. For the same reason, other students often continue to wear dark sunglasses in the classroom.

Interestingly, I find that these Irlen Syndrome-affected students are frequently unaware of how sensitive they are to artificial lighting conditions, and they are equally unaware of the relationship between this sensitivity and their dislike of reading. Similarly, when I ask my students if a classroom's fluorescent light bothers them, a large percentage raise their hands (for one of my student surveys for Irlen Syndrome, see Graph B on pages 40-41). When I have numerous students who dislike the classroom's fluorescent lighting—provided the classroom has adequate natural lighting from windows—I will turn off the overhead fluorescent lighting and leave it off. At times when I try to turn the lights back on, students will protest. It is rare that any of the students request the fluorescent lighting be turned back on.

I am frequently surprised that students are not aware of how much they are affected by light sensitivity. For example, a student sent to me for evaluation responded when I asked her about light sensitivity, "I don't think that I am sensitive to light." However, when this student took the Irlen screening instrument, "Reading Strategies Questionnaire," she marked nearly every question indicating extreme and frequent visual distress. When I placed an appropriately-colored transparency over reading material, this student's response—like so many others—was an immediate exclamation, "Oh, my God! That's so much clearer; I can read the page much more easily now!" Then she turned to me and asked, "Isn't that easier for you to read too?" I often hear this kind of an exclamation, along with students asking me if I, too, can now see the page more clearly and read what is written more easily. Students assume that if this color overlay clarifies the printed page for them, then it must do the same for me. However, the color of overlay that works for one student may not work for another—or for me.

Of course, this student assumption regarding the power of colored overlays to clarify print underscores why Irlen Syndrome has been slow in finding acceptance in some institutional settings. Those who suffer from Irlen Syndrome believe that everyone sees the printed page as they do, and those who do not have this visual-perceptual problem assume that everyone sees the printed page as they do, that is, without distortions and light-induced strain. In addition, students are not aware of the ways in which Irlen Syndrome handicaps their comprehension of what they read. Another of my students was not aware that Irlen Syndrome was affecting her ability to correctly decode questions on multiple choice tests. Once I had screened her and found that she did have Irlen Syndrome, she shared this insight: "Now I understand why I sometimes misread and answer test questions incorrectly; I read 'hostile' when the word was 'holistic' and, as a result, I marked the wrong answer." Certainly, students cannot read accurately when they perceive that the letters and words are bouncing around on the page and appear blurred, indistinct, or washed out.

This latter problem of erratically-moving eyes was described to me by one of my students who took her daughter for Irlen screening. My student's daughter was to begin college soon, and my student had heard me speak about Irlen Syndrome and recognized that her daughter probably was affected. After a screening that did indicate a moderately severe case of Irlen Syndrome, my student took her daughter to an Irlen diagnostician to discover the correct color for tinted lenses. A few days later, my student arrived in a state of happy excitement and described her daughter's diagnostic session to me: "When my daughter tried to read without an appropriately-colored overlay," she recounted, "I watched her eyes and noticed that they were bouncing all over the page. When the Irlen diagnostician placed the right color transparency on the printed page, I could see my daughter's eyes moving smoothly along each line and then down to the following line. It was quite an amazing transformation." My student was delighted to have discovered her daughter's "invisible" reading barrier, and now she felt certain that her bright and motivated daughter would be able to meet the challenge of college-level work.

Many educators are not aware that Irlen Syndrome is a common stumbling block for student learning. When educators do become aware of Irlen Syndrome, they may discount its importance or significance for learning difficulties. These educators need to know that over the past two decades, research studies in U.S. universities and abroad have explored the incidence and causes of Irlen Syndrome, as well as the effectiveness of Helen Irlen's remedial interventions. Fortunately for affected students, Irlen Syndrome is becoming better understood by many educators; some are learning that the effectiveness of the Irlen Method of remediation has been validated by new and exciting research.

For example, research conducted by the U.S. Navy at Stanford University, along with research carried out at the University of Utah, has demonstrated that Irlen Syndrome is real and constitutes a serious barrier for affected students (Irvine, 2005). Additional research involving brain scans has demonstrated impressive improvement in brain functioning when an individual seriously affected by Irlen Syndrome wears appropriately tinted lenses or uses a colored transparency (Amen, 2005; Dobrin, 2005). Researchers in Australia and England, as well as in the U.S., have conducted controlled studies with students of the Irlen intervention and reported impressive results: Students' reading levels have improved dramatically within short periods of time when they have been provided with the appropriately-colored transparencies (Noble et al., 2004; O'Connor et al., 1990; Robinson & Foreman, 1999). Irlen Syndrome interventions are now recognized and permitted on achievement tests in several states, including California, Massachusetts, and Washington State.

Step 2. Remediating students' auditory-processing problems

For students whose primary reading and learning problem is auditory-processing dyslexia, that is, an inability to connect the sounds of letters and words with their written forms (inability to connect phonemes to graphemes), my Basic Program suggests computer exercises based on research conducted by Rutgers University's Prof. Paula Tallal and her colleagues (Tallal, 1993; Tallal et al., 1996). Prof. Tallal and her associates have discovered that computer programs that slow down—stretch—speech sounds allow dyslexic students with auditory-processing problems to more easily connect phonemes to graphemes. Similarly, Earobics is a computer program of exercises that assist students in making the necessary connections between sounds and text. With these exercises, students' brains learn to make the missing connections in ways more similar to the brains of non-dyslexic students. The Earobics program can be found online at www.earobics.com and has been recommended to me by professors at Washington State University's Speech and Hearing Center.

Dr. Paula Tallal and other researchers have founded Scientific Learning, a company distributing brain-based systems of remediation for dyslexic persons to educational institutions and learning professionals. Scientific Learning's specialists have developed the Fast ForWord "stretched" speech exercises, along with other exercises based on Dr. Tallal's research. Dr. Tallal and other leading dyslexia researchers, Dr. Sally Shaywitz, for example, have discovered that some dyslexic brains have a problem making the connection between the sound of letters and the sight of letters. This is the essential *phoneme* (letter sound) to *grapheme* (letter symbol) connection. By using computers to lengthen the time that the brain is exposed to the sounds and sights of letters and words, dyslexic individuals can begin to build more exact neural models of letter sounds and words in their brains. Some researchers have hypothesized that some dyslexics may experience difficulty making this phoneme-grapheme connection because of their genetic inheritance.

These researchers posit a genetic slowness in nervous impulse transmission along certain speech and reading pathways called "magnocellular" pathways in dyslexics' brains. These pathways function at a faster pace in normal readers. Because magnocellular pathways are found in several brain regions, research may eventually support their slowed functioning as implicated in several types of dyslexia.

Scientific Learning's Fast ForWord programs, although effective, are only available to educational institutions and professionals. I'm informed, however, that the Earobics program can accomplish similar results if used extensively, and this program is available to parents for home use.

Dr. Tallal's computer-modulated and "stretched-speech" method has had good success in helping struggling readers become more successful. Therefore, parents whose children are severely affected by dyslexia may want to consult Scientific Learning's website: *www.scientificlearning.com* for more information about this method and allow their children to access the excellent demonstrations of the various reading exercises. By having their children experience these online demonstration exercises, parents may gain insights into some of the specific auditory-processing difficulties with which their children are struggling (Tallal, 1993; Tallal et al., 1996). In Chapter Four, I outline how teachers could institutionalize my Basic Program—and certainly parents could lobby their local schools to obtain and make available to struggling students the brain-training software that *A Practical Guide* recommends.

This *Guide's* Basic Program uses the knowledge gained from Drs. Shaywitz and Tallal's research to present a brain "rewiring" program based on the human brain's ability to learn at any age. Brain plasticity research demonstrates that even adults learning English as a second language, or students from families that did not value or stress language and reading, can still improve the way their brains function. Cognitive scientists have found that students' "dyslexia" problems may stem from the lack of preliteracy experiences in infancy and early childhood. I've found that many of my English-as-a-second-language students were never literate in their first language.

For whatever reason, even if students did not develop phonemic awareness in early childhood, and even if they were lacking in this awareness and other preliteracy skills when they began school, they still can gain brain power by identifying their invisible barriers and by following the computer exercises recommended in this chapter. These computer exercises have been developed by scientific researchers to produce better brain "wiring," that is, the more exact neural models and systems essential for better attention, memory, and reading fluency and comprehension.

Most parents will know if their child is falling behind in reading and can assess their child for Irlen Syndrome dyslexia. This visual-perceptual form of dyslexia is often accompanied by problems in the auditory-processing modality as well. To find out if students need to use some of these auditory-processing program interventions, parents certainly can speak to their children's teachers to determine if their children are reading on grade level. Children who are falling behind or who have already fallen behind should be assessed for both Irlen Syndrome and auditory-processing dyslexia.

Bright children who are only minimally to moderately behind their peers' reading level may have unidentified visual-perceptual and/or auditory-processing difficulties that can be rapidly remediated by means of colored overlays and/or the "ear-training" exercises provided by the Earobics software program. My Basic Program of remediation is presented at the end of this chapter. I further address these cognitive-processing problems in Chapter Four when I provide preventive reading / learning strategy suggestions appropriate for younger (preschool and early elementary) students whose parents or older siblings have struggled with learning difficulties and who may already be showing signs of these difficulties.

Step 3. Improving students' ability to pay attention

Many educators and cognitive neuroscientists are concerned with the problem of teaching and motivating the growing number of American students who have problems staying focused on their school work, paying attention in the classroom, following directions, and completing homework assignments. Cognitive neuroscientists have conducted research to discover if the ability to pay attention can be improved through training. Preliminary research results have demonstrated that, given the plasticity of the human brain at every age, attention is an ability that can be improved, especially with the use of specially-designed computer software exercises (Posner, 2004; Posner & Rothbart, 2005; Posner et al., 2003).

If parents have identified a problem with their children's ability to pay attention by using Dr. Daniel Amen's free assessments presented in Chapter Two, then they will be happy to learn about the inexpensive software programs that have demonstrated that attention is a trainable skill. Much scientific research is still needed to gain an understanding of the degree to which attention can be strengthened in the brain, but preliminary results from Dr. Michael Posner of the Sackler Institute for Developmental Psychobiology and the University of Oregon are encouraging. Dr. Posner's research studies demonstrate that the brain's neural networks responsible for focus, attention to stimuli, and maintaining attention can be strengthened. He also has stated that if, as his research shows, training attention is possible, then training attention abilities should become an important educational objective for all students. Sustaining focus and attention are keys, according to Dr. Posner, for student proficiency in high-level skills. Prof. Posner has stated that his work on remediating children's attention abilities should be considered "not just as remediation but as a normal part of education. Attention plays a very important role in acquisition of high-level skills, and if attention is trainable, it becomes attractive for preschool preparation" (Posner, 2003, pp. 58-9). My pilot studies with older children and with my adult students also have demonstrated that attention can be improved in a relatively short time.

Therefore, if parents have used Dr. Amen's assessments and identified their child as minimally or moderately lacking in attention and focus, then parents can acquire Parrot Software's effective attention and memory-strengthening exercises. In fact, even if parents believe that their children's attention and focus abilities need much improvement, I still recommend that their children begin their program of remediation by working with Parrot Software. The best Parrot Software exercise program for building attention and focus is that of "Hierarchical Attention Training," a program that provides numerous attention-building activities within a range of difficulty. These exercises not only build focus and attention abilities, but are also designed to help students learn to inhibit their tendencies towards impulsive behaviors.

If parents have identified learning problems that can be helped by the Irlen colored overlays and/or listening exercises, such as those of Earobics, they may find that these interventions coupled with the Parrot Software attention-building exercises are all that their children will need to become effective readers and learners.

A Practical Guide's Basic Program, provided at the end of this chapter (along with the sample programs presented in Appendixes B[1]—B[5]), will get children started on the path towards effectively identifying and remediating those crucial visual-perceptual, listening, and attention abilities that need strengthening in so many of today's students. In addition, because educational researchers find many students deficient in their working-memory abilities, I will next address two critical components of working memory, namely, visual working memory and auditory working memory.

Step 4. Improving students' working memory

Few are the students who are satisfied with their memory abilities. Working memory, also called short-term memory, is often cited by students as the weak link in their memory systems. Many students complain that they have to work extremely hard to retain what they are reading or hearing long enough to comprehend, process, and move the information into their long-term memory stores. "If I can just manage to grasp the information I am reading or hearing, hold onto it long enough to make sense of it, then I can get it into my long-term memory. Once I've done that," students will tell me, "then I have a much easier time recalling information and using this information to move on to more difficult concepts." In fact, researchers have noted that problems in basic cognitive-processing mechanisms in the brain (for example, problems in processing letters, sounds, and words) are often related to working-memory problems (Robbins, Mehta & Sahakian, 2000).

Students who struggle with Irlen Syndrome's visual-perceptual difficulties and who battle their brains' tendencies to wander and lose focus, frequently complain that they can't remember what they have just heard or what they have just read. Even students who do not have visual-perceptual difficulties or problems with attention or focus can be failing academically because of working-memory problems. I want to share with parents a story that illustrates how just one cognitive-processing weakness can defeat even an excellent mind.

Soon after beginning my Washington State community college teaching assignment, I began to notice large numbers of students with cognitive-processing difficulties. These students' difficulties have motivated my learning programs and inspired this book's Basic Program. One day towards the beginning of the academic year, I was sitting at my desk preparing for class when an older gentleman suddenly appeared in my office doorway. I thought that he must be a book salesman and because I only had a few minutes before my class began, I tried to tell him, politely, to leave. This dignified and earnest man was, I soon learned, a school psychologist working on some of the same student cognitive-processing problems that I had identified as presenting difficulties for my students.

I grew to know and respect this man as a colleague over a span of about four years, during which time we collaborated and shared notes on student learning difficulties. This gifted Ph.D. told me that he had had enormous problems learning in school. One day when we were discussing student learning, he confided to me, "At one point I had the opportunity to look through my high school files, and I found that my teachers had evaluated me and marked my files with the words, 'Not College Material.'" I was surprised to hear this news and curious to learn more because my professor friend had written several books on learning, developed learning programs, and taught many subjects at all levels, including graduate school. "How did you manage to obtain your doctorate with such a history of school failure and such a discouraging prediction?" I asked.

My colleague chuckled and explained that towards the end of high school he had begun to realize that he had a severe weakness in his auditory working memory. "I could not for the life of me remember anything that I heard," he said. "Information was literally in one ear and out the other! However," he continued, "once I had understood what my problem was, I began to carry a notebook with me everywhere. I wrote down everything right away, learned to take good notes in class, and from that time forward it was all As and Bs, all the way to my doctorate in psychology from the University of California, Santa Barbara."

This story inspired me then, just as it had inspired my colleague, to look for ways to help other students who, like himself, had intelligence and abilities that were blocked by significant cognitive-processing weaknesses. I had realized, as my colleague had realized, that these invisible barriers to learning could be minimized, or even removed, if only they could be identified. Like my colleague's experience, many students find that their central learning problem involves working memory, whether auditory working memory or visual working memory—or, as is frequently the case, both. Increasing working-memory capabilities, my colleague and I found, can make the difference between failure and success for many students.

For help strengthening children's working memory in both the auditory and visual modalities, I recommend two Parrot Software computer programs:

- *Visual & Auditory Memory Span*
- *Word Memory and Discrimination.*

These programs were developed by Dr. Frederick Weiner, a former speech pathologist at Pennsylvania State University, in conjunction with clinical specialists who worked with individuals experiencing memory, attention, and reasoning deficits. Dr. Weiner founded Parrot Software in 1981, and has seen his over 60 programs used with great success in many hospitals and rehabilitation centers throughout the United States, including Veterans Administration Hospitals, Kaiser Permanente, the National Rehabilitation Hospital, HealthSouth Rehabilitation Centers, and the University of Michigan Hospital, as well as in educational institutions. Additionally, these programs are used in international centers and have been translated into five languages.

The *Visual & Auditory Memory Span* exercises will provide children with a good assessment of their working-memory capabilities in these two modalities. It can also rather quickly help children increase their working-memory span, that is, the number of remembered elements in both modalities. The *Word Memory and Discrimination* program will help children with working-memory capabilities and with listening skills, as well as strengthening their ability to pay attention and focus. These programs have already proven themselves effective in rehabilitation communities, but I and other educators have also had success using them with students from middle school through college.

Exercises like these very effectively helped college students in a Washington State Department of Social and Health Services program developed for the State's Welfare-to-Work population. Furthermore, the Director of California's Community College High Tech Training Units informed me that California uses Parrot Software programs, along with others in my Basic Program, to develop memory and attention abilities in California's struggling community-college students. In short, these Parrot Software programs, along with many others the company has developed, have a long and impressive track record of helping brains overcome weaknesses in memory, attention, and reasoning.

One example of Parrot Software programs' effectiveness totally surprised me. One of my college students, a bright and motivated young adult with ADHD and very poor auditory-memory skills, asked me for help. I set up a schedule for her, using the Parrot Software auditory memory-strengthening program. This student had complained of not being able to remember what she heard in class and, therefore, she taped her professors' lectures. I knew that she had been working on these memory exercises for many hours when she came running up to me one day quite excited. Holding out her notebook, she explained that she had continued to tape her professors' lectures, but one day her tape recorder broke in an especially difficult lecture-only class. "I panicked," she reported. "I told myself, you are dead!" But then she recounted how she decided to take notes despite her anxious state of mind. "You see," she ended triumphantly, "it works! I was able to take four complete pages of good notes—something I had never been able to do before!" The student held out her notebook for me to examine, and she had, indeed, written four well-organized pages of notes. To make her case even stronger, this student showed me a page of notes she had taken before completing the memory-strengthening exercises. These pages looked like the chicken scratches of a beginning elementary school child. Even I could not believe the difference!

I cannot guarantee that all students will experience such outstanding improvement in their working memories and note-taking abilities. This student was highly motivated and determined to improve her areas of weakness. However, with equal motivation and willingness to spend the required time practicing, I do believe that students will find themselves improving beyond what they or their parents thought they could accomplish.

When I first began my university career at the University of California, Los Angeles, one of my professors commented, "Most people can do much more than they realize; they just never try, and so they never do the things that they are truly capable of accomplishing." My experience working with students, with identifying their areas of strength and of weakness—and, especially, my experiences remediating students' cognitive-processing weaknesses—have taught me this UCLA professor was entirely correct. Students don't know how much they can accomplish, how much they can improve, until they try. My experience has been that students who try do succeed. My years of work with students with learning "differences," coupled with my knowledge of the brain's "rewiring" capabilities, convince me that all students will be surprised at what they can accomplish—if they will only try (Swanson, 2000; Verhalghen, 2004).

By now, parents will have identified the areas of their children's brains that need strengthening. Next, parents can help their children follow the suggested Basic Program's exercises at the end of this chapter so that their children will become more effective readers and learners. However, before turning to the end of this chapter, let's consider one final aspect of reading and learning, an aspect that constitutes the foundation for reading, indeed, for all thinking and learning.

Step 5. Improving students' vocabulary levels

Thus far, we have considered problems of physiology (students' anxious bodily responses to examination stress), and we have examined learning problems related to students' brain "wiring," specifically, problems with students' visual-perceptual, listening, attention, memory, and other brain-based cognitive-processing abilities. Parents have learned how their children can combat test anxiety and then access free online cognitive-processing assessments. Most importantly, I have stressed that by learning first to identify and then to remediate their children's specific problems with cognitive processing, parents will eliminate much of the test anxiety their children have experienced in the past. The final ability essential for children's success in reading and learning is children's ability to understand and use words: I have found that most students' vocabulary levels need improvement.

I address word power last, but word power is far from the least of the abilities students need to succeed in the classroom and, eventually, in the workplace. I also address word power last because, judging from my teaching experience and research, most students who are struggling readers and learners, suffer from the hidden handicaps of visual-perceptual and / or auditory-processing dyslexia, ADHD, and/or poor working memory. *These problems require identification and remediation first and foremost.*

Of course, some students may not harbor any of these invisible handicaps but, instead, are struggling in school because they are recent immigrants for whom English is a second language. Many others come from poverty-level backgrounds where parents have not had the resources in time and money to provide academically enriching experiences for their children. Many parents are not aware of the critical importance of speaking to a preverbal infant who, by hearing language, becomes verbally proficient in lasting ways. Many parents are not aware of the critical importance of reading to their children while they are still infants and toddlers.

Unfortunately, some children experience neglect and, at times, even abuse. Often, these poverty-level or working-class students had parents who wanted to be good parents but whose own abusive parenting backgrounds, low educational levels, and stressful lives made good parenting nearly impossible for them. Parents who were not read to as children may not realize the importance of reading to their infants and young children. Parents who are exhausted by the enormous stresses of working two or more minimum-wage jobs may not have the energy to spend "quality"—or any—time with their children.

For all of these reasons, educators today are concerned that a substantial percentage of American students do not read much, and some do not read at all. Without extensive and intensive experiences with reading often and widely, many working-class or poverty-level students enter elementary school with only half or less of the word power of their middle-class peers. Research has linked such lack of vocabulary skills with lower high school graduation rates and lower lifetime earnings (Biemiller, 2001; Chall & Jacobs, 2003; Hart & Risley, 2003).

Once children have begun strengthening their cognitive-processing abilities, the next most important ability for them to strengthen is their ability to recognize and understand words. The Johnson O'Connor Foundation's 70 years of research on word power conclusively showed that vocabulary abilities are linked to school and job success. Research and teaching experience have taught me that large numbers of my college students, as well as the younger students like Danny, whom I have tutored, do not have the word power required by their textbooks. This statement will not be disputed by most college and university professors, or by elementary and high-school instructors. In fact, professional journals in the fields of education and cognitive psychology are filled with research documenting and lamenting entering college students' lack of preparation in basic math and English skills. Remember the Gallup Organization survey cited earlier that discovered an alarming drop in the average American 14-year-old's average vocabulary from 25,000 words in 1950 to only 10,000 words in 1999. Even Ivy League universities have high percentages of students who test into "developmental" math, English, and reading courses. For example, WordSmart, the vocabulary-building software program I recommend, is used in such prestigious universities as Purdue and MIT in their remediation courses (Bowker, 1977; Wood, 2001).

Even if parents believe that their children's vocabulary levels are sufficient for the school and work tasks they expect their children to encounter in life, I am betting that their children would sail through these tasks with less effort and more success by simply increasing their word power. Remember my University of California, Irvine, professor who told us graduate students, "In any discipline, learning the lingo is 90 percent of the battle." I have seen bright students from middle-class backgrounds, students who showed no evidence of learning disorders, do poorly on multiple choice tests because they did not know the simplest words. As mentioned, students have asked me to define simple words such as "precede," "accomplish," and "autocratic." Not knowing these words meant that the students could not figure out the correct answers to exam questions. Not knowing these words—and many other elementary, high school or college-level words—means that these students must struggle to understand even the simplest textbook.

Recognizing the abysmally low vocabulary levels of today's non-reading students, some of my most distinguished colleagues in psychology have written texts with "dumbed down" vocabulary and with many words defined in the main body of the text. Such texts are welcome, of course, because they are helpful to immigrant students, to students from the lower socioeconomic levels, and to students with hidden learning problems. I have tackled the problem of my students' impoverished vocabularies by stressing at the beginning of each course the need for them to purchase a good vocabulary workbook—and to spend a few minutes every day increasing their word power. The book I have recommended is *Word Power* published by the Kaplan Institute (Schneider, 2001).

Some of my students have taken my advice and given their fellow classmates and me feedback on their results. One student, for example, was taking a second course from me and she interrupted me as I was making my sales pitch about vocabulary-building books and exercises. Her story is worth repeating: My student told the class, "I took Dr. Morrow's advice and bought *Word Power,* and I used it frequently to learn prefixes, suffixes, and the roots of words. The next quarter, I was really excited to discover that I could understand a lot of what the professors were talking about even when I didn't know all of the words my professors were using. I found that I was able to grasp the main ideas because I could figure out what many of the new words meant—and reading my textbooks was a lot easier, too!" This student, along with many others, became enthusiastic supporters of my learning program, helping me to run pilot studies in the local schools.

For many years I had screened vocabulary-building software because I knew that all students would benefit by increasing their word power. Finally, I found what I believe to be the best program on the market, a program with decades of research supporting it and a money-back track record of helping students pass high-stakes tests. This program is *WordSmart,* the diagnostic and vocabulary-building software program that uses the huge empirical database gathered by Johnson O'Connor, the father of aptitude testing.

A Harvard-trained polymath, Johnson O'Connor became head of electrical engineering for GE, where he led research into aptitudes and appropriate job placement. Through his Foundation's 70 years of research, testing over a million subjects, O'Connor found evidence supporting the link between individuals' vocabulary levels and their academic and workplace success. His research developed the vocabulary-learning principles that are the foundation for WordSmart's effective computer software programs. Utilizing O'Connor's extensive research into vocabulary acquisition, WordSmart guarantees that only 20 hours of exercises will raise students' SAT verbal scores by 100 points or more. The O'Connor Foundation research provides evidence that better word knowledge results in better reading abilities, better thinking, and greater school and career success.

One of my WordSmart-trained students wrote the following about her experience with this vocabulary-building software exercise program: "The WordSmart program was fun and informative. When I returned to school [after the summer break], I would say a word that I had no clue I was going to say. Then I would realize, oh, OK, that's WordSmart talking. I even had a couple people ask me for coffee to discuss my ideas about politics. I only had an eighth grade education before I went to get my GED. Now I want more of WordSmart [because] if this is what happens with only a few lessons . . . I can, and do, relate to college-level persons." This student—like so many others with significant learning difficulties—discovered the joy of learning through WordSmart and the other brain-building exercises in this *Guide*'s Basic Program.

Review of the Basic Program

The abilities that I have listed in this book are those key abilities indispensable for students' success in every life arena. These skills work together to ensure children's capabilities *to know* and *to grow* more effective as students, and to become life-long learners able to improve—at all ages—their relationships with friends and family. Like so many educators before me, I have discovered that helping students achieve academic success can eliminate students' test anxieties, as well as raise their self-confidence levels and self-esteem. Finally, succeeding academically enables students to eliminate self-defeating behaviors brought about by their invisible barriers to reading and learning.

Here, now, are the assessment and remediation steps summarized so parents can guide their children to the academic and personal success they deserve.

Note: *For detailed assessment steps to aid in identifying their children's hidden barriers to reading and learning, parents can refer to Chapter Two, pages 79-81.*

Review of Assessments

Consult the following websites:

1. www.wwcc.edu/student_services/online_adv/success/test_test.cfm for questionnaire identifying symptoms of test anxiety in students (site is maintained by Walla Walla Community College, www.wwcc.edu);

2. www.irlen.com for visual-perceptual difficulties caused by Irlen Syndrome, and www.earobics.com for auditory-processing problems;

3. www.amenclinic.com to identify problems with attention and maintaining focus;

4. www.parrotsoftware.com to identify students' memory and other cognitive-processing problems; and

5. www.wordsmart.com to obtain information about students' vocabulary levels.

Review of Remediation

After following the Basic Program's steps for assessing and identifying their children's learning problems, parents will be able to more effectively implement a remediation plan using the following steps:

Step 1. Remediating visual-perceptual processing difficulties (Irlen Syndrome dyslexia): If the child has some degree of Irlen Syndrome, parents should consult www.irlen. com to locate a trained Irlen screener who can assist them in finding the right color transparency for their child. For children severely affected by Irlen Syndrome, parents can consult this website to locate trained Irlen diagnosticians in their area. These diagnosticians are experts in finding their child's correct color in tinted lenses.

It is important that parents realize that the best color in a transparency to lay over reading material and computer screens may not be the best tint for reading lenses. Helen Irlen's colored transparencies and tinted lenses are used all over the world by hundreds of thousands of people of all ages to reduce or eliminate the physical symptoms (fatigue, migraines, stomachaches when reading or doing computer work) and the dyslexia symptoms (blurring of text, rereading, misreading, inability to keep eyes tracking smoothly along the lines, and lack of reading comprehension) that accompany Irlen Syndrome dyslexia.

Step 2. Remediating auditory-processing difficulties (phonological dyslexia): Visual-perceptual and auditory-processing problems are often—although not always—present together. After remediation for Irlen Syndrome, if needed, parents should consider if their child has weak listening skills resulting in difficulties with pronunciation and with connecting the sounds of letters and words to their written forms (an inability to connect phonemes to graphemes). These are some of the central symptoms of auditory-processing dyslexia. Excellent "brain rewiring" computer software exercises are available using the Earobics program and can be found for home use at www.earobics.com. These solutions are very reasonably priced.

Step 3. Improving children's ability to pay attention: If parents have identified problems with their children's attention abilities, then I believe that the most effective and reasonable software on the market for alleviating these difficulties can be found at www.parrotsoftware.com. I especially recommend "Hierarchical Attention Training." If a child has severe problems with attention, then Parrot Software's online diagnostic will indicate other attention and concentration programs that are also effective. Parrot Software's website includes demonstrations of all software programs.

Step 4. Improving children's working-memory abilities: Parrot Software exercises are especially effective if parents have discovered through the Parrot Software diagnostic that their children's working-memory capabilities need strengthening. I have used with great student success the "Visual and Auditory Memory Span" exercises. For students who have memory, attention, and concentration problems, Parrot Software's "Visual and Auditory Memory Span," along with "Word Memory and Discrimination" and "Hierarchical Attention Training" programs are excellent and inexpensive choices. An Internet version that provides access to all Parrot Software programs is available for $24.95 per month (www.parrotsoftware.com).

Step 5. Improving children's vocabulary levels: WordSmart is, in my opinion, quite simply the best vocabulary-expanding program on the market. Additionally, it comes with a money-back guarantee if students' test scores do not increase significantly (see the website for details). WordSmart's programs are packaged for grade-school children (first through fifth grade), middle-school children (fifth through ninth grade), high school children (ninth through twelfth grade), as well as for adult learners. Parents can go online to find more information about WordSmart at www.WordSmart.com.

> Note: *Any prices quoted may be subject to change—with programs costing less or more—at the discretion of the software companies. Parents can check current prices on the companies' websites. Also note that software companies may change their websites to improve customers' access to their products.*

Suggested Remediation Program

Once parents have assessed their children for barriers to reading and learning, they will have identified the primary stumbling blocks that have been preventing their children from working up to their full academic potential. Parents will then be prepared to set up a program of remediation for their children based on the information provided in this chapter. To assist parents in setting up such a program, I am providing the following: (Note: *Parents should also see the sample programs presented in Appendixes B^1– B ^{5}*):

1. If students have been identified with Irlen Syndrome, they should use the colored transparency most effective for them over their computer screen as they work on their remediation exercises.

2. On Monday through Friday, most students should complete 10-15 minutes of "Visual & Auditory Memory Span" (Parrot Software). Parents should focus on their children's weakest cognitive-processing modalities, namely, visual or auditory processing. Students can be taught how to increase the level of difficulty as their proficiency increases. Typically, as students' proficiency increases, so will their motivation. By competing with themselves to improve, students soon become caught up in the game of improving their abilities and seeing their scores increase.

Students who have special difficulties with their listening skills (connecting the sounds they hear with the letters they see) should complete 10-15 minutes a day of the auditory delivery of "Word Memory and Discrimination" (Parrot Software), or choose the Earobics exercises designed for their age group (www.earobics.com). Earobics is not an expensive program, but it is a very effective one for auditory-processing dyslexia. To keep students challenged and interested, especially if they have problems maintaining their attention, "Word Memory and Discrimination" exercises can be alternated with the exercises mentioned above.

3. On Monday through Fridays, most students should complete 20-40 minutes of WordSmart's vocabulary-building software exercises.

Parents need to develop flexible but consistent exercise programs based on their children's ages, responses to the various exercises, and the severity and number of their children's learning problems (Parents should refer to sample programs in the appendixes).

Parents should note that I am developing a Basic Program website that will help them set up the most effective exercise program depending upon their individual child's specific barriers to reading and learning.

Here are the WordSmart exercises listed in the order in which students should complete them:

(1) Flash cards: Learn word origins and synonyms. This exercise can be omitted for younger children and for children with more than moderate degrees of attention problems. For English-language learners and students who struggle with vocabulary deficiencies, the Flash Cards exercise is especially helpful.

(2) Multiple choice: Choose the correct synonym.

(3) Column matching: Match the word with the definition by moving the word to column on the right.

(4) Sentence completion: Find the word to complete the sentence or phrase and type it.

(5) Laser review game: Play the "video game." Students of all ages love this game that motivates them to work their way through the previous exercises.

The WordSmart Program has been scientifically designed, developed, and tested to teach vocabulary contextually so that students of all ages will move their new vocabulary words from their short-term working-memory into their long-term memory stores. WordSmart will automatically move each student up to the next level provided the student scores from 70 percent to 90 percent correct, depending on the specific exercise. Periodically, WordSmart retests the student before moving the student to a higher level. Should the student not have retained the proficiency necessary for retaining the word groups in long-term memory, then the program automatically moves the student back to the previous level of proficiency. In this way, long-term memory storage of vocabulary is assured.

What's ahead

In Chapter Four, I present parents with the early signs that their very young children may be experiencing reading / learning difficulties. In addition, I present modifications of this Basic Program for preschool and early elementary school-age children. Chapter Four also includes suggestions for parents and for teachers so that educational institutions can set up a computer learning lab with the Basic Program's software.

Suggested reading

Brubaker, C. L. (2005). *L. D. from the inside out: A survival guide for parents.* Casper, WY: Whiskey Creek Press.

Robertson, I. H. (2000). *Mind sculpture: Unlocking your brain's untapped potential.* New York: Fromm International.

Sternberg, R. J., & Grigorenko, E. L. (1999). *Our labeled children: What every parent and teacher needs to know about learning disabilities.* Cambridge, MA: Perseus Publishing.

Tobias, S. (1995). *Overcoming math anxiety.* New York: W. W. Norton.

Travis, J. (1996). Let the games begin: Brain-training video games and stretched speech may help language-impaired kids and dyslexics. *Science News, 149,* 104-106.

CHAPTER FOUR

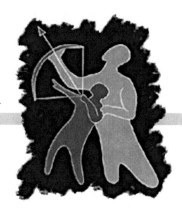

Setting up the Basic Program
Part I—For parents

How to help young children thrive emotionally and academically

The importance of emotional intelligence for learning

Parents of young children from preschool age through early elementary school would be well advised to read the two books on emotional intelligence listed as suggested readings at the end of this chapter. Of course, these books would be helpful reading for the parents of any age student. Why a child's EQ—the child's emotional intelligence—matters as much as IQ for that child's learning is well explained in Prof. John Gottman's book, *Raising an Emotionally Intelligent Child* (1998), and in Daniel Goleman's book, *Emotional Intelligence* (1995). Gottman and Goleman both emphasize how the positive interactions that infants and toddlers have with their caregivers provide young children with a solid nervous system and "emotional basics," fostering optimal learning on all levels. Goleman calls these basics a good "heart start" and states that school readiness depends as much on a child's emotional capacities as on a child's intellectual capabilities. Moreover, children who do not have self-confidence, self-control, and the ability to get along with others will not fulfill their potential for learning, according to these experts' research (Goleman, 1995; Gottman, 1998).

Children who are chronically stressed may even experience damage to their brains' learning and memory centers. Children who appear anxious in everyday situations and who are afraid to try learning new skills, such as throwing a ball, climbing a jungle gym, riding a tricycle, or pouring their own milk, may have unhealthy and brain-damaging levels of stress hormones. Therefore, it is especially important for parents to learn about young children's developmental norms. Knowledge of developmental norms and their variability will teach parents that wide differences exist in children's readiness to learn various motor, language, and intellectual skills. Expecting too much of a young child creates stress for that child; however, young children, even very young children, are much more competent and ready to learn than child development experts previously thought.

Given the importance of eliminating chronic anxiety and the stresses that may have generated this anxiety, parents of very young children would be wise to visit the test anxiety website listed in Chapters Two and Three. By selecting and answering the age-applicable test anxiety questions, parents can investigate whether their children are experiencing unusual degrees of anxiety in challenging (testing) situations. Even very young children can be afraid to try something new if they feel they may fail. This reluctance to expose themselves to failure may also reflect the hidden learning problems that are more prevalent than most parents and educators realize and that the Basic Program is designed to identify and reduce or remove.

Therefore, when a child of any age is lagging far behind peers and classmates, these developmental lags should signal parents that invisible stumbling blocks to learning that require identification and remediation may be present. My teaching and research experience have demonstrated that it is never too late to intervene and help students toward more effective learning. I have helped students in their 50s and 60s improve their memory, attention, and general learning abilities. However, early appropriate intervention is always preferable to waiting until students have accumulated a history of failure and the low self-esteem that accompanies that failure.

Although preschool and elementary school teachers can help parents decide if their children's worrisome behaviors (for example, restlessness, impulsivity, aggressiveness, and inattention) are related to learning difficulties, parents are the best observers of their children. Parents have been observing them since birth. As with my cousin's son Danny, problematic nervous systems announce themselves very early—sometimes even before birth. Children who are slow to walk and talk may not go on to have problems learning to read, but parents can encourage their children's speaking and preliteracy skills by playing "point and name" games, reading to them, and playing rhyming games with their children. Preschool children who have trouble rhyming, with the alphabet, and with the alphabetic principle (learning the sounds of letters) may be at risk for dyslexia (Biemiller, 2001; Hamilton & Glascoe, 2006).

Children with rhyming and alphabet letter sound problems could benefit from the cognitive-processing software recommended in this chapter. Recent cognitive neuroscience research has demonstrated with brain imaging that even dyslexic brains' faulty "wiring" can be changed for the better (*Science News*, 2001, *160*, p. 155; Shaywitz, 2003). Furthermore, recent language acquisition research conducted by psycholinguists with infants and very young children suggests that children with Specific Language Impairment (SLI)—namely, children who have difficulties communicating in words and sentences—may have "a broader deficit in underlying learning mechanisms" that require a targeting of "the cognitive skills that underlie language, rather than focusing exclusively on a child's language impairment." (Cynkar, 2007, p. 46). *A Practical Guide*'s Basic Program does help children build essential cognitive-processing skills. Therefore, computer games and exercises that improve very young children's ability to hear and distinguish sounds, and to connect these sounds with letters and objects, may improve the phonological skills that are critically important as children begin learning to read (Tallal et al., 1996; Travis, 1996; Wood, 2001). Parents can help their very young children grasp the concept of the relationship between sounds and letters, practice playing rhyming and naming games with them, and provide them with access to the computer software programs recommended by this book. In this way, parents can ensure that their children's brains are properly wired with essential pre-reading literacy skills.

Moreover, growing evidence from the neurosciences, as well as from educators, supports the effectiveness of focusing on building fluency in the basic components upon which reading and learning mastery depends (Willingham, 2007; Johnson & Layne, 1992). Exceptionally bright children, like Danny, may harbor multiple reading barriers and yet not exhibit these difficulties until high school or college where remediation in basic skills is not emphasized. In high school or college, these bright students may finally be diagnosed with learning "disabilities," but instead of receiving remediation help, these students are only supplied with "accommodations" in the form of more time on tests or note takers in class. These accommodations are helpful; however, it would be far better if these students were provided with interventions that capitalize on the brain's ability to rewire itself at any age (Catone & Brady, 2005; Murray, 2000; Robertson, 2000; Robertson & Murre, 1999).

Although remediations can be effectively applied with older students, voluminous research supports prevention and remediation at the earliest ages. Certainly, the new knowledge upon which this *Guide's* Basic Program rests is not yet widely understood by educators (Elmore, 2005). Most educators do know, however, that failing to remediate children with hidden learning barriers comes at the high cost of rising school dropout rates, particularly among boys, and the unacceptable rates of addiction, delinquency, and suicide among our youth (Coles, 2004; Daniel et al., 2006; Lauerman, 2001; Lyon, 1998; Winters, 1997).

Finally, before turning to the assessment and remediation of cognitive-processing problems that may lead to learning problems in very young children, I urge parents whose children are exhibiting any of the difficulties mentioned to have these children's hearing and vision carefully checked. Parents should keep in mind, however, that visual-perceptual dyslexia, i.e., Irlen Syndrome, is essentially unknown to most optometrists and ophthalmologists. These specialists test patients' eyes in dimly lighted rooms where light sensitivity will not become apparent (Gillespie, 2001;

Levine, 2003; Remick et al., 2000; Whiting, 1994-95). In addition, problems with vision and hearing may interfere with children's ability to pay attention and to stay on task once they enter school. Early diagnosis is also essential for children with attention problems. The neuroscience research news here, too, is encouraging: Children's brains can be retrained; moreover, supplying nutrients essential for young children's rapidly growing brains can in some cases control hyperactivity as effectively as medication (Harding et al., 2003; Stevens, 2000; Stevens et al., 1995).

Although intellectual giftedness coupled with academic learning problems—the problems of "twice exceptionality"—have not been extensively studied, I do suspect that many gifted children are not challenged to achieve their full potential because they are compensating "well enough" and achieving at an "acceptable" average level (Schwartz, 2007, p. 94). Educators are aware that gifted students need intellectual challenges or they may succumb to boredom and drop out of school mentally. Less well understood is the danger of gifted students physically dropping out of school because of the painful conflicts they face when unidentified learning difficulties cause them to fall far short of their considerable learning potential.

Finally, parents who themselves struggled with reading in school, whether or not they were identified as dyslexic, need to observe their young children's sound production and discrimination, along with the length and complexity of their children's sentences. Preschool children from families with dyslexia have a greater chance of struggling with reading once they begin school. About half of students who have exhibited problems speaking and pronouncing correctly do go on in preschool and early elementary grades to experience reading difficulties (Hamilton & Glascoe, 2006). Similarly, parents with a history of attention deficits, serious memory problems, or light sensitivity also need to be alert to signs of these problems in their very young children.

How to modify the Basic Program for young children

Parents can modify the Basic Program for their preschool or early elementary school-age children using the following steps:

Step 1. *Identifying and remediating visual-perceptual dyslexia in young children*

Parents can access Helen Irlen's website (www.irlen.com) and identify whether their child has the physical symptoms of Irlen Syndrome. For a child who has not yet learned to read, symptoms that indicate light sensitivity may warn that some degree of Irlen Syndrome is present. Even very young children can be screened to discover the best color transparency to place over computer screens when the children play games or do brain-building exercises. Nowadays, children of two and three are becoming computer-literate. The glare from a computer screen may be especially bothersome for children with Irlen Syndrome. Of course, parents can start by darkening computer screens and by changing the screens' background tones. Parents can observe how long children stay in front of the screen and whether they express physical discomfort either in words or by restless body movements. In this way, parents can gauge whether the computer screen adjustments have relieved their children's discomfort.

Again, families in which some members already have been identified with Irlen Syndrome's light sensitivity or other symptoms of dyslexia should be especially alert to their preschool children's nonverbal behaviors because, like other reading difficulties, Irlen Syndrome dyslexia appears to have a strong genetic component (Lyytinen et al., 2001; Robinson, 1997).

For the young child who appears to have some degree of Irlen Syndrome, parents can experiment with different colored sheets of paper on which the child can draw, paint, or practice letters and numbers. If children are in preschool, kindergarten, or early elementary school, parents can suggest to teachers and caregivers that worksheets, or playsheets, be provided in a number of different colors. Children can be encouraged to choose the colored sheet that they like best. One of my former students is presently teaching in a local elementary school and doing research for her master's degree in education. Her master's thesis research involves providing Irlen Syndrome children with spelling, math, and other subject worksheets printed in different colors. The colors provided are those that children commonly prefer, for example, blue, blue-gray, gray, peach, green, and purple.

When I last spoke with her, my student had not yet completed and published her research, but she has reported to me that the differences in academic performance of the Irlen-Syndrome students are quite amazing. For example, one third grader's printing of his name on high contrast white paper looked more like the work of a preschool child barely able to print. When my student provided this third grader with a choice of colored worksheets, he was immediately able to print his name so well that the results compared favorably with older children's printing ability. My student cited another example involving math worksheets: Another of her third graders was working hard but was only able to calculate the right answers to two or three (out of about 20) problems when the problems were high-contrast black print on white worksheets. When this third grader was provided with a choice of colored worksheets printed with the same math problems, she was able to correctly solve 15 or 16 problems out of 20. Indeed, huge academic improvements can occur by simply providing children with a choice of colored worksheets, along with the usual, high-contrast black print on white paper. Irlen-Syndrome children will choose the colored worksheet that best helps them successfully complete the required task.

One of my colleagues who is a certified Irlen screener has informed me that children as young as first graders can be screened for Irlen Syndrome, even though they are not yet readers. Helen Irlen's website provides the locations of screeners throughout the U.S. This website also provides an online assessment that can indicate to parents if their child is a candidate for a complete Irlen screening. Parents can save their children much heartache and frustration if Irlen-Syndrome problems are identified early and the effective and inexpensive colored transparency interventions are provided. I am presently working with several college students who are severely affected by Irlen Syndrome. Each of them has expressed gratitude for my having identified the source of their learning difficulties, and each has stated they wished their Irlen-Syndrome dyslexia had been identified and remediated early in their school years. "I could have been saved so much failure and frustration," each of them confided to me.

Many of my college students have brought their elementary or high-school age children to me for pre-screening and identification of Irlen Syndrome. One of my college's staff members, "Martha," asked me to screen her teenage daughter, "Janice," for Irlen Syndrome. Martha was concerned about her daughter's reading difficulties, especially because her daughter was about to enter college. Janice, indeed, did demonstrate a high degree of Irlen Syndrome on Helen Irlen's "Reading Strategies Questionnaire," so I referred her to an Irlen screener for further evaluation. A few days later, Martha came to share Janice's experiences at the screening. Martha was very pleased and excited by what she had observed: "I noticed that Janice's eyes were bouncing all over the page as the screener presented her with various reading materials," Martha reported. "But when the screener found the right color transparency and placed it over the reading materials, Janice's eyes suddenly moved smoothly along each line of print, and smoothly down to the next line. I was amazed by this transformation in her ability to effortlessly track along the printed lines and down the page!" Janice told her mother, "the words stopped moving around when the overlay was placed on the page." As follow up, I asked Martha a few weeks into the college term how Janice was doing, and Martha informed me that her daughter was enjoying her college work and had reported that reading her school texts was less stressful and more enjoyable than ever before.

Younger children will not be as aware of the stress caused by their sensitivity to light, and they may not be able to articulate well the difference that colored overlays make in their enjoyment of close work. That is why parents will need to observe carefully the body language of their preschoolers when they are presented with close work of any kind, whether computer games and exercises, or coloring- and-pasting activities.

Parents can also observe the lighting preferences of their young children: Do their children want to work in dim light? Do they rub their eyes and squint when watching TV or playing video games? Young children with severe Irlen-Syndrome problems may avoid many visual activities and not want to "read" along when parents are reading children's story books to them.

If this is the case, then once children severely affected by Irlen Syndrome begin to read, they may benefit greatly by having lenses tinted in the color that works best for them. Certainly, children should be screened by a qualified optometrist or ophthalmologist and fitted, if necessary, with corrective lenses. If corrective lenses are needed, these glasses can be tinted in the appropriate color to remove, or at least diminish, Irlen Syndrome visual-perceptual dyslexia. No other coatings should be applied to the corrective lenses so that the color tint can be applied.

Although many young children, along with some adults, will not be aware of their sensitivity to light, even some early elementary school children are quite aware of this sensitivity. Recently, a former colleague introduced me to her six-year-old granddaughter who was experiencing difficulties learning to read. This cute, big brown-eyed first grader, "Sally," could shyly indicate her answers as I read Helen Irlen's "Reading Strategies Questionnaire." I soon realized that Sally was, indeed, quite affected by Irlen Syndrome. When I showed Sally various colored transparencies, she was readily able to indicate a color that made reading more comfortable for her. Knowing that it was important to provide Sally with precisely the correct color, I referred her to a certified Irlen screener. My colleague called me later to report her granddaughter's progress and the family's delight at discovering the source of Sally's school difficulties. I was not surprised to learn that Sally required three transparencies, two turquoise and one purple, laid one on top of the other. Sally was quite severely affected and needed much muting of glare to read comfortably.

Step 2. *Identifying and remediating auditory-processing dyslexia in young children*

Young children who have a type of auditory-processing dyslexia may not be identified as early as might be desired. Because there is good research evidence that many, if not most, of the stumbling blocks to reading and learning have a genetic component, parents may want to take preventive measures if either one or both of them—or one of their parents—had dyslexia. One of the first students in my earlier college learning program was failing her difficult dental hygiene classes. "Deena" was, in fact, about to be dismissed from the program. Because she was hardworking, likable, and clearly intelligent, the Head of the Dental Hygiene Program asked me to identify Deena's problems and, if possible, remediate them. I soon discovered that Deena was quite dyslexic and that she had great difficulty remembering how to sequence and order items—a serious problem for someone who must be responsible for laying out dental instruments and for preparing equipment and medication needed for administering dental anesthesia.

I set up a program for Deena, and she worked hard on her assigned memory and sequencing exercises. When she retook the learning assessments, these abilities had significantly improved. After completing the remediation exercises that I had assigned her, this highly dyslexic student passed all of her courses, graduated, and went to work as a dental hygienist. A few years later, I received a call from Deena who wanted more program information so she would be prepared to work with her children. "My husband is also dyslexic," she informed me, "and I know that our children will probably have some problems as well." Deena's inquiry revealed her intelligence and foresight. She realized that with both of their parents struggling with dyslexia, her children would need careful observation and the preventive measures that I am suggesting for preschoolers and early elementary- school-age children. I was happy to provide Deena with advice for recognizing signs of developing learning problems, along with suggestions like those in this book for preventing, or at least remediating, problems as they arose.

This brief anecdote reveals a recurring theme well-known to learning specialists: When children demonstrate reading difficulties that reflect cognitive-processing problems, there is a high probability that a parent, grandparent, or other relative will have demonstrated similar problems in school. Therefore, parents who are aware of their own or other family members' learning difficulties, particularly a dislike of reading, need to be especially observant of their young children's early learning behaviors. By intervening before their children have fallen behind their peers, parents will prevent much of the frustration, dislike of school, and low self-esteem that accompanies children's reading failures. Students who are falling behind may develop stomachaches, want to stay home from school, and refuse to participate in group or individual oral reading activities.

Dr. Sally Shaywitz's book, *Overcoming Dyslexia* (2003), is a valuable resource for parents who are anticipating, as was my student, that their children may have inherited auditory-processing dyslexia. Dr. Shaywitz describes the early symptoms of serious auditory-processing dyslexia whereby children have difficulty learning the "alphabetic principle," namely, that letters printed on a page are linked to sounds. Dr. Shaywitz also describes how children may have difficulty understanding rhymes, or blending and segmenting the letters in simple words taught in the early grades. For families severely affected by auditory-processing dyslexia, I recommend investing in Dr. Sally Shaywitz's text, while observing children for signs of visual-perceptual dyslexia that may also cause physical symptoms such as headaches and stomachaches, along with school phobias and test anxiety.

There are, in fact, a number of enjoyable, simple, and inexpensive computer software programs that can help children whose families harbor "dyslexia genes." In Chapter Three, I mentioned a program that works well for young children, namely, Earobics. Earobics (www.earobics.com) is modestly priced and quite effective for training children's ears to connect sounds with visual images and symbols. Furthermore, Parrot Software has programs designed to improve children's listening skills. Especially valuable is Parrot Software's *Perception of Sounds* program, appropriate for young children who have begun to read simple text. Depending upon the ability level of the children, Parrot Software has other programs for young children that will strengthen faulty cognitive-processing systems involving memory and attention, and thereby prepare children for greater reading success. Among these programs are *Visual Attention Tracking* and *Auditory and Visual Picture Recognition* (for nonreaders). Parents can go online at www.parrotsoftware.com and take for their young child the "Communication Survey" which is a diagnostic questionnaire and then explore the excellent demonstrations of programs suggested. Parents may want to have their children experience the demonstration exercises to observe the ability of the children to do the exercises and how well the exercises engage and hold their children's interest.

The specific learning problems of each child will help parents decide which brain-building programs are needed; the child's age, patience, and other personality characteristics, as well as the child's specific learning problems, all need consideration when parents are deciding how to set up their child's exercise program. Appendix B[5] at the end of this book presents a bar graph template that parents can fill in to provide them and their children with a quick visual approximation of learning strengths and areas that require remediation; also provided is a suggested exercise program. Parents can refer to the suggested practice schedules (days and times for appropriate exercises) provided by Chapter Three's Basic Program (pages 104-110). They should also examine the sample learning difficulties profiles and sample remediation exercises provided in Appendixes B[1]—B[4].

While more time spent practicing the appropriate brain-building exercises is better than less time spent, parents must be sensitive to the preferences of their children. Children should enjoy doing these exercises. The software has been designed to be fun and to give children a sense of improved cognitive functioning. When I asked one of my older students if he could feel improvement in his thinking processes, he commented, "Oh, yes. I do feel that my memory and ability to read are improved by the exercises you assigned me, but I just don't have the words to express what I'm sensing."

He paused for a moment, and then he exclaimed, "I think that my synapses are firing much better!" My student had actually found just the right words! In Appendix C, I have provided a date and time schedule where parents and children can keep track of the specific software exercises used, along with the amount of practice time spent each day.

A Basic Program exercise website is planned and should be available to parents and children in 2008.

Step 3. Identifying and remediating young children's inability to pay attention

Each of the reading and learning problems identified and remediated by *A Practical Guide's* Basic Program interact with every other. These interaction effects mean that a child who is seriously affected by Irlen Syndrome may have problems paying attention and may avoid reading whenever possible. The avoidance of reading, in turn, means that the child may not be gaining grade-level vocabulary and certainly will have problems remembering what is seen and heard. Most research into learning difficulties has reported that many children with one brain-based cognitive-processing problem harbor other problems as well. Certainly, serious visual-perceptual and auditory-processing problems will negatively impact children's ability to pay attention, their working memory, and their vocabulary-building capabilities.

Young children, especially boys, who have problems paying attention and who are impulsive and "hyperactive" may be identified as having Attention Deficit Hyperactive Disorder (ADHD) and may be prescribed medication for this learning difficulty. Often, young girls who are not paying attention may not be identified as having ADHD because they are not causing the classroom disruptions that characterize hyperactive young boys. Parents need to consult with physicians who are qualified to diagnose ADHD or ADD (attention deficit without hyperactivity) in young children. Not all pediatricians, even those who profess knowledge of dyslexia, are qualified to diagnose the various subtypes of ADHD. Such was the case with Danny's ADHD problems;

Nan chose his pediatrician because he was a specialist in treating children with dyslexia. Unfortunately, this specialist knew nothing about attention problems and Irlen Syndrome. Nan thought that Danny could be hyperthyroid, and she knew that hyperthyroidism and allergy problems, which Danny also had, could cause symptoms of inattention. This pediatrician dismissed Nan's concerns, and Danny went well into his twenties before another doctor did, indeed, diagnose his malfunctioning thyroid.

Parents also must keep in mind that very bright children can exhibit some ADHD or ADD symptoms which may simply be caused by boredom, accompanied by the young child's high energy levels and nervous system immaturity. An additional complication can occur when an ADHD child is a gifted child—which was the case with Danny (Hartnett et al., 2004). In my experience, above-average intelligence and problems with attention are linked more often than parents, teachers, and physicians realize. Furthermore, parents should keep in mind that visual-perceptual and/or auditory-processing dyslexias can cause or contribute to children's problems paying attention.

Parents can begin to identify problems with attention deficits, even in very young children, by accessing Dr. Daniel Amen's website: www.amenclinic.com. Dr. Amen has provided an exceptionally useful ADHD-subtype assessment questionnaire that parents can answer on behalf of their young child. By responding to this questionnaire, parents can obtain invaluable information regarding whether their child is possibly—or probably—harboring one or more ADHD subtypes. In addition, Dr. Amen's website provides indispensable diet, exercise, natural supplement, and medication information linked to each ADHD subtype. Again, identifying and remediating problems with attention as early as possible in a child's academic career can make the difference between that child's success and failure. Dr. Amen's website also makes available information about his many books on the brain-based learning problems that can handicap students of all ages, along with information about how to recognize and reduce these problems.

Dr. Amen's newsletter, "Brain in the News," is archived, with past issues available on his website. This helpful newsletter, to which parents can subscribe free of charge, provides the latest information on treating brain-based problems with natural substances, foremost among them the omega-3 fatty acid fish oils. In Chapter Five, I discuss natural supplements that university research studies indicate will alleviate some of the symptoms of ADHD and ADD, while supporting optimum brain performance for students with other learning difficulties.

Step 4. *Assessing and remediating young children's memory and other cognitive-processing problems*

Preschool and early elementary school-age children who have been identified with visual-perceptual and/or auditory-processing dyslexias and/or attention deficits will benefit greatly from computer software games and exercises that strengthen their visual and auditory working-memory skills. Chapter Two recommended that parents check out Parrot Software's website, www.parrotsoftware.com and have their older students take this website's excellent brief diagnostic questionnaire ("Communication Survey"). Although this questionnaire may be of limited utility for very young children, parents can visit this site and learn about the abilities that Parrot Software exercises can effectively remediate, and they can experience the cognition-strengthening exercises through the demonstrations available. Furthermore, parents can answer the questionnaire for themselves and experience the website's demonstration exercises. In this way, they can gain insight into familial patterns of strengths and weaknesses, as well as insight into capabilities their young children might benefit from strengthening. Two of the Parrot Software programs that will be helpful for young children's listening skills are *Visual Attention Tracking* and *Auditory and Visual Picture Recognition* (for nonreaders).

There are many computer software games for young children, but the advantage of the Parrot Software program exercises is the targeting of specific cognitive-processing deficits. By focusing remediation exercises on one area at a time, the Parrot Software exercises can help young children overcome their present cognitive-processing weaknesses and head off future learning difficulties.

Step 5. *Assessing and remediating young children's vocabularies*

Researchers investigating learning differences have found that there are many reasons why children may develop reading difficulties and avoid reading. This book discusses some of the most common problems. The visual-perceptual (Irlen Syndrome) and auditory-processing dyslexias can cause problems with attention, as well as the avoidance of reading that results in impoverished vocabularies. Children from families where reading is not emphasized, or where the language used at home is not English, can also have impoverished English vocabularies by the time they enter kindergarten. If a child does not understand much of the language spoken in school, for whatever reason, then that child will not grasp and retain in memory the grade-level concepts that teachers present. It is essential, therefore, that parents read to their children from infancy onwards, and play naming games with their toddlers and preschool children on a daily basis in the supermarket, at the park or zoo, and around the house and garden (Allen & Sethi, 2004; Chall & Jacobs, 2003; Hart & Risley, 2003).

This book has recommended the vocabulary-building software programs of Word-Smart, www.wordsmart.com, for students from about age eight through adulthood. For very young preschool age and struggling early elementary age children, WordSmart has developed an effective phonics program. Over many decades battles have raged between reading experts advocating "whole language" approaches to reading and those insisting on a "phonics-first" approach. Most recent research, however, does support the need for solid phonics instruction for most children (Shaywitz, 2003; Tallal et al., 1996). WordSmart's phonics software is uniquely designed to prepare preschool children for early reading success in kindergarten and early elementary school.

By providing their young children with a fun and effective phonics pre-reading program, parents offer some preventive protection for their children who may be genetically predisposed to develop reading difficulties caused by auditory-processing dyslexia. Of course, parents should remain alert to the possibility that their children may—also or instead—have problems with visual-perceptual processing (Irlen Syndrome) and observe if their children appear to be especially light sensitive. This latter problem would require the interventions and remediations previously discussed. If children's reading and learning difficulties are identified and remediated early, evidence is emerging from the brain sciences that their difficulties, whether caused by genetic "glitches" or lack of exposure to literacy skills, can be overcome by "rewiring" of their brains (Shaywitz, 2003; Tallal et al., 1996).

Parents may want to encourage their local schools to provide this Basic Program of assessment and remediation to all students as needed. Certainly, all students could benefit from improved working memory, attention, and vocabulary.

What's ahead

This book's final chapter addresses some of the other important steps involving appropriate exercise and healthy diet that parents can take to help their children overcome their academic struggles and succeed in the classroom and beyond.

Part II—For educators

The Basic Program in educational institutions

Note: *The Basic Program may also be helpful for business training institutes, vocational rehabilitation companies, and correctional facilities.*

Why the Basic Program will help "power up" students' brains

Widespread failures in U.S. elementary and high-school education have led to increasing rates of illiteracy, unemployment, welfare dependency, and incarceration. In recent years, educators have expressed concerns about the increasing number of students entering higher education with poor basic skills, attention deficits, and learning "disabilities."

U.S. poverty rates are high, with nearly one in five children living below the poverty level. Because low-income parents tend not to speak or to read much to their children, research has shown that up to 30 million fewer words have been heard by low-income children on average by the time they reach three years of age as compared to children from more affluent families (Hart & Risley, 2003). By the time these children enter kindergarten, their vocabularies are only one-half or less as large as the vocabularies of their middle-class peers. Other research reports that one in five high-school graduates are functionally illiterate and "cannot perform such everyday tasks as reading bus schedules or determining the correct change for even small purchases" (Roueche & Roueche, 1999, p. 1). Many other studies have reported that the majority of unwed mothers are illiterate, as are the majority of Americans—adults and juveniles—who are arrested and incarcerated (Maloney, 2003; Winters, 1997). In this context, it is interesting to note that Dr. Sally Shaywitz's research studies have found that as many as one in five students are affected by dyslexia (Shaywitz, 2003).

Studies of juveniles arrested and jailed find that as many as 90 percent have visual or visual-perceptual processing problems. Other studies of inmates in our correctional institutions report that over 75 percent have learning "disabilities" such as those discussed in Chapters One and Two (Winters, 1997). Loss of manufacturing jobs and on-the-job injuries propel older workers into vocational rehabilitation or academic retraining programs. These workers often need to upgrade their literacy skills for a high-tech job market. Community college instructors frequently find that workers returning to school for retraining have significant learning difficulties that were not identified when they were in elementary school. Because of their lack of academic success, these workers opted for jobs in trades, construction, or manufacturing. The loss of family-wage jobs in these sectors means that workers in retraining programs must look to jobs in information technology or other high-skill areas, or risk finding no job at all. If these workers' learning difficulties are not identified and remediated, the jobs that they do qualify for—if they can find one—will barely maintain them and their families above poverty level.

Losses to national productivity caused by low levels of literacy have been estimated at over $225 billion per year. Without additional programs designed to find and help these injured or retraining workers—especially those with learning difficulties—national productivity losses will continue to escalate. Without effective programs designed to identify and remediate all students' learning difficulties, the high-tech jobs that do pay family wages will continue to be unfilled—or outsourced.

Meanwhile, confidence in the predictive value of standard IQ tests has decreased, and awareness of multiple intelligences—and learning differences—has increased (Sternberg, 1999, 1996). These new understandings, coupled with research supporting the brain's ability to learn at any age, open educational doors for older students who require retraining. They also present opportunities to locate and help students when their brains are most "plastic" and malleable in the early grades. In addition, despite the well-documented "Flynn Effect" of IQ scores rising throughout modern societies, student achievement levels, especially in basic skills, have been sinking. As a result, more and more developmental courses are required for entering and returning college students (Neisser, 1998; Perkins, 1995). Educators at all levels are searching to understand these contradictory findings and to develop effective means to help students of all ages master basic skills. Foremost among these skills is reading proficiency.

Aside from high poverty rates and high immigration rates of non-English speaking people, educators often blame low literacy rates on a failure of present generations of students to read. They blame too much TV watching and too many extracurricular activities, including part-time jobs, that occupy time spent by earlier generations in reading activities. Educators also fault pressures on instructors at all levels to lower standards and socially promote students, thereby releasing students from pressures to learn.

The increasing pressures on educators

Certainly, the causes of America's high illiteracy rates are complex. However, today all U.S. educational institutions are charged with the unprecedented task of improving literacy rates at all educational levels. The challenges of a global marketplace and a shrinking planet demand that our citizens become competent, life-long learners. In response, federal legislation has mandated that "no child [be] left behind," and businesses are increasing their post-employment job training programs.

Standards-based education and high-stakes testing, criticized by many experienced educators, have been government's solutions to the crisis of American educational underachievement. At the same time, legislators in my Washington State are questioning the need to fund "developmental" courses for college and university students. They argue that students should have reached college levels in math, English, and reading upon graduation from high school—or the high school diploma means nothing. I cannot argue with this logic. However, educators cannot easily move from the "is," the status quo, to the "should." Our country's high rates of immigration, our need to help large numbers of working adults retool for new careers, and the increasing requirements for higher levels of education to meet the job demands of a high-tech world—all of these factors make "developmental" and supplemental educational programs more essential than ever before.

All of the problems that I have briefly outlined here are undoubtedly familiar to most professional readers of this chapter. Whether instructors teach in an elementary school, middle school, high school, or in higher education, or whether they teach in a business training program, in vocational rehabilitation programs, or in our nation's correctional facilities, they have had personal experience with the problems I have listed. They, like me, have undoubtedly thought about solutions to our country's critical educational problems. They, like me, have undoubtedly tried many new approaches and programs that they thought might help their students achieve higher levels of literacy, become better readers and more effective learners. Depending upon their institutional setting, they have undoubtedly been caught between their students' desire for high marks and their own desire to maintain standards. Within our nation's K-through-12 schools, pressures on teachers from parents and administrators are also intense and conflicting. What to do? they ask, as do I. *A Practical Guide*'s Basic Program is my response to the American illiteracy crisis and represents an effective way to remove many barriers impeding student learning and, thereby, raise students' academic achievement levels.

Is technology the cure for low literacy rates?

Technology is often seen as providing solutions for low student achievement. But technology in the form of the Internet and computerized learning programs can be a double-edged sword. Students can use technology to cheat as well as to learn. Often students are more technologically astute than their teachers. They can go online to purchase completed term papers; they can copy information from websites without citing the source—so now plagiarism is also a growing problem for most instructors in middle schools, high schools, and colleges. One of the Western Psychological Association conferences I attended a few years ago took student cheating as its main theme, with a featured presentation that asked, "Are we in American education producing lemons?"

Many of my college colleagues have revised their writing assignments to make plagiarism more difficult. Still, students do find ways to plagiarize. Proving that students have plagiarized is time-consuming for teachers. Even when students are caught "red-handed," they will often deny knowing that what they have done is cheating (at my college, instructors have the onus of proving "intent"), and students will complain to administrators about instructors who charge them with plagiarism. School administrators typically do not want any trouble from irate parents, nor do they want the bad publicity that can come their way from such parents. The "my-child-would-never-knowingly-cheat" claim has made headlines in some states and has cost educators their jobs. In higher education, administrators have begun to see students as "consumers" or "customers," and, as the saying goes, "the customer is always right."

"Distance" education, also touted as another technological solution to educational dilemmas, provides more opportunities for cheating. It further distances educators from face-to-face interactions with students. "Distance" education over the Internet can saddle educators with the burden of providing 24/7 tutoring services individually to students enrolled in their Internet courses. These are just some of the problems technology and Internet access have caused educators.

I do believe, however, that technology can solve some of these thorny educational dilemmas. This book's Basic Program shows parents and students how to use the Internet to find free assessments and identify brain-based learning difficulties. The Basic Program utilizes computer technology to show parents, teachers, and students how to develop individualized exercise programs designed to "rewire" students' brains and eliminate their most important stumbling blocks to reading and learning proficiency.

I have been a believer in and an early adopter of new learning technologies—but a *highly selective* adopter. I am confident that technology offers many solutions to our problems as educators, but we must remain alert and choose carefully what we do adopt, and be judicious as to how we adapt our selections for our students.

Over many years of teaching, I have noted that the students most likely to plagiarize or to cheat in other ways are students struggling with language, reading, and learning difficulties. Of course, some students have absorbed from our culture, or their subculture, the idea that education is for "nerds" and not an asset that they care to work for. However, I think that we are at a turning point in American society when the diminishing number of family-wage jobs and the requirements of high-paying jobs, along with the increasing costs of a higher- education degree, are awakening many students to the realities of our twenty-first century global village. These wakeup calls are not yet heard by all, but the calls are growing louder and they are not going away.

This awakening is good news for educators. I am encouraged by our national focus on education and by the many new programs, technologically based or not, now vying for educators' attention. In fact, many of us are overwhelmed by all of the demands such programs place upon us to keep up and revise our lesson plans and assignments. I am certain that many of these new programs and educational initiatives will transform American education, provided there is a weeding out of those that don't work. However, we educators need to ask ourselves, "Does American education have enough time to work through all of these new ideas before we lose the global race to gain and retain the best-paying jobs?" And, "Are we putting enough resources into the right places?" These questions are being debated in educational and public-policy circles and will be debated for some time to come.

I think that selective adopters of evidence-based programs—programs like this *Guide's* Basic Program—will bring these new approaches based on cutting-edge cognitive neuroscience research and technology into our schools, businesses, and the many other American institutions dedicated to increasing our nation's intellectual capital. I predict that these evidence-based programs will raise literacy levels across our nation within a very few years.

How to set up the Basic Program at an educational institution

Whether the institution is a school, college, business training program, or correctional facility, it is essential for instructors to educate the institution's administrators— especially those in charge of the purse strings—about the Basic Program's low cost and learning effectiveness. Instructors must be absolutely certain that they have their administrators' support and, if they work with other instructors, those educators should be brought on board as well. I speak from experience, having set up, or assisted in setting up, many learning programs. Educators, especially those working with at-risk students, are almost always excited to learn about the possibilities of rapidly "rewiring" students' brains to improve their visual-perceptual and auditory processing abilities, along with their attention, memory, and vocabulary skills. Before addressing an institution's instructors, I make sure I have first presented my programs to a given institution's administration. Given the growing governmental pressures on teachers and administrators to leave no child (or adult) behind, and in spite of the underfunded status of NCLB, I am finding a growing receptiveness to *A Practical Guide*'s Basic Program.

Despite the recent media attention to the latest neuroscience research about the human brain's "plasticity" and ability to respond to appropriate interventions with new "wiring," even well-informed educators have many questions about these new approaches to learning. A few years ago, I presented an earlier computerized learning program to community college educators at the prestigious National Institute for Staff and Organizational Development (NISOD) Conference sponsored by the University of Texas, Austin. I had been invited to give a preconference seminar entitled, *Multiple Intelligences: Helping All Students Achieve Success in Learning.*

My learning program presentation was extremely well-received, with standing room only and a long line of enthusiastic educators waiting to ask further questions when I had finished. The urgent need felt by educators for this kind of assessment and computerized remediation became apparent to me at this conference. The questions and concerns raised by my professional audience about institutionalizing a Basic Program bear repeating and answering here.

Questions about setting up the Basic Program

Question (Q): You have spoken about students' "multiple intelligences" and "learning-style differences." If I have 40 students in my class, how can I teach to 40 different learning styles?

Answer (A): "Multiple intelligences" and "learning styles" refer to different but overlapping concepts. Research carried out by Harvard's Prof. Howard Gardner and Yale's Prof. Robert Sternberg shows that there are many ways that students can be intelligent and that not all of the "intelligences" make for academic success, or "school smarts." Prof. Sternberg, for example, has shown that practical and creative intelligence are as important for life success as analytical intelligence; the latter is more specifically helpful for success in academic settings (Eisner, 2004; Gardner, 1983; Sternberg, 2001, 1996). Precise relationships among intelligences, learning styles, and learning differences still demand more research, but certainly there are a limited number of intelligences and learning styles. The Basic Program is founded on research that identifies and indicates how to remediate the most common reading and learning difficulties experienced by students of all ages.

It is well known that some students are visual learners, some are auditory learners, and some learn best by doing, and so on. Most students have a preferred learning style, but most students also are capable of learning in other modalities, although perhaps not as easily. New research indicates that the *content*, rather than the student's learning style, should determine the modality of presentation (Willingham, 2005).

> *Rather than a focus on learning styles, the focus of the Basic Program is on developing students' weaker intelligences and expanding the ways in which students can access and process information. That is, the Basic Program works to expand students' learning styles. When the ways in which students can learn are increased, then they can adapt more easily if instructors' teaching styles are not meshing with their preferred learning style.*

Of course, most instructors do realize the importance of supporting their lectures with visuals and, whenever possible, with hands-on demonstrations of concepts. In addition, most individuals, whether teachers or students, learn best when facts and concepts are presented in a variety of ways and with examples that speak to their own life experiences.

Q: How are learning styles related to the abilities that the Basic Program targets for improvement?

A: There is a direct relationship between students' preferred learning style or styles, and their strongest cognitive-processing ability or abilities. It is easy to understand that a student who is a good auditory learner will prefer to learn through lectures. Conversely, as is the case with so many students today, students who cannot easily process information presented auditorily will prefer to learn through seeing or doing. Students with Irlen Syndrome have problems with visual-perceptual processing. They may learn to read fluently if their processing problem is mild, but they must put forth much more effort than students without this problem. This fact, of course, means that visual learning is difficult for them. If these same students are good auditory learners, then they may compensate up to a point. However, in our modern technological society, reading well is an indispensable ability, so Irlen Syndrome students benefit greatly from colored overlays or tinted lenses.

Similarly, students may have difficulties with auditory processing: They may have problems connecting the phonemes—the simple sounds that they hear—and the graphemes—or letter symbols—that they see in written text. These students, like Irlen Syndrome students, will have difficulty with reading. In fact, students often struggle to process information in *both* the visual and auditory modalities.

Therefore, it is important to remember that there are many cognitive-processing problems that contribute to reading and learning weaknesses, and that most students harbor more than one cognitive-processing difficulty. Furthermore, these processing difficulties can range from mild to severe. Learning problems are complex and a long way from being fully understood. However, the assessments that the Basic Program recommends will provide parents and educators with knowledge about areas to target for intervention. Visual-perceptual (Irlen Syndrome) and auditory-processing dyslexias, along with ADHD, working-memory problems and vocabulary deficits, are all common invisible barriers to reading and learning success, and many students struggle with several of these problems at the same time.

It is most important, however, that parents and teachers understand the rapidly accumulating cognitive psychology and cognitive neuroscience research detailing how students' brains can be rewired and their "intelligences" increased by appropriate teaching and technology (Perkins, 1995; Posner, 2004; Posner & Rothbart, 2005; Sternberg, 2001, 1999).

In short, the Basic Program has shown that targeted interventions can rewire students' brains and alleviate their specific learning problems. Improved student learning will, in turn, significantly raise literacy levels in American society.

Q: You have mentioned a few software programs for remediation and the need to screen and remediate students for Irlen Syndrome. What are the costs involved with implementing the remediation portion of the Basic Program?

A: The Basic Program is very cost effective because most of the remediation is done with low-cost computer software. Of course, the school or training facility must have computers, along with tech support capable of keeping computers functioning. Tech support is also available at the two software companies I recommend, namely, Parrot Software and WordSmart. Computers are becoming more commonly available to students at all of the sites where learning takes place. Also essential is at least one (but preferably more) staff person, depending on the number of students, who understands learning problems and recognizes that computer exercises can rewire students' brains. Students struggling to overcome their learning difficulties need supportive and caring people around them while they are working. This staff person or persons can easily be trained to screen students for Irlen Syndrome. The colored overlays for students who need them are inexpensive, about $3 to $5 per overlay, depending on the quantities in which they are ordered.

The Parrot Software site license is $500 for institutions (no site license charges for home computer use), and most of their programs run about $100. The WordSmart software Volumes A through E (the volumes most needed by elementary school age children and adults to raise their basic vocabulary levels), including site license, starts at $2500, based on school criteria such as student enrollment, which volumes are needed, whether computers are PC or Mac, and whether staff development is purchased. The consumer (home version) of WordSmart is not licensable for classroom use. Instructors should note, however, that the classroom version is much less expensive per child and features many tools and benefits neither necessary, nor available, for home use. The assessments that identify many learning problems are free online. Most important for the individual learner, WordSmart has a website for learning centers that can be accessed as much as desired by one learner for one year at the reasonable cost of $50 per student, provided twenty students subscribe to the service. As mentioned in Chapter Two, students with severe dyslexia and/or ADHD problems may need other programs, such as Earobics for auditory-processing dyslexia (Note that these prices may be subject to change and may be somewhat less or more than the quotations provided here. Parents and teachers will need to check the companies' websites for up-to-date pricing information.)

One of the important strengths of the Basic Program is its effectiveness in helping all students learn, even those without obvious learning problems. All students—especially elementary and middle-school age children, but also adults needing basic skills remediation—can benefit from vocabulary development and from work to increase their working memory and attention spans. Like chicken soup, as one of my colleagues used to say, this program can't hurt anybody! In fact, my pilot study data indicate that the Basic Program can help significant numbers of students struggling with reading and learning to achieve greater academic success.

Q: What have your pilot study data shown?

A: The college students in my pilot study gained, on average, nearly four grade levels in reading with only 25 hours, on average, of remediation exercises. Note that all of these pilot study students were affected by Irlen Syndrome and were using the appropriately-colored transparencies over their computer screens and over their reading materials. These pilot study college students had also been diagnosed with other cognitive-processing difficulties, such as ADHD and auditory-processing dyslexia. My middle-school age pilot study students have gained—with an average of 24 hours of remediation exercises over six weeks—from one year to five years of grade level in reading. These sixth- and seventh-grade students all had Irlen Syndrome and most were English-as-a-Second Language students in a poverty-level after-school tutoring center.

Q: What are the steps in setting up the Basic Program?

A: The six steps to setting up the Basic Program are as follows:

Step 1. Introduce the Basic Program to the institution / facility: The Basic Program can be introduced as a course, as supplemental instruction for a course or program of study, or it can be set up as a pilot study for a small group.

If an institution or training facility wants to gather experimental data with a pilot study that tests the Basic Program's effectiveness, then students, and the parents of underage students, should sign consent forms to participate in the program. These consent forms will explain what the study is designed to do and what advantages the study should bring them. For a sample consent form, see Appendix D. By signing the consent form for a pilot study, students and/or parents are agreeing to 24-25 hours of remediation over a period of six to eight weeks. Shorter programs of 20 hours over five weeks should also bring significant results for most students.

Step 2: Instruct students about learning differences and barriers to learning: This essential step involves an orientation session that educates students, depending upon their age and level of understanding, about learning differences, brain plasticity, and the need to identify any invisible barriers to learning that they might have. In my research and experience, I find that most students who are struggling with reading and learning are highly anxious about their abilities. They secretly fear that they are "stupid" and can't learn. They may have developed elaborate, self-defeating behaviors. Many have either become the class clown (males, more typically) or withdrawn into wallflower status (usually females).

Therefore, giving students information about how they may have been misled or mislabeled is a first giant step towards motivating them to participate in identifying what has slowed their learning progress. Students must be convinced that their invisible learning barriers, once identified, can be eliminated, or at least greatly reduced. Communicating these understandings helps students to believe in themselves and encourages them to do their best on the remediation exercises.

It is especially important to communicate to students that everyone has learning strengths and weaknesses, that having a learning weakness does not make them less intelligent, and that most learning weaknesses can be reduced or eliminated through concentrated effort on the Basic Program's exercises. Gaining knowledge about their individual learning strengths is also helpful. To this end, there should be discussions to raise students' level of awareness about how information is accessed and processed.

Step 3. Assess students: Students are assessed on the following instruments:

a. Irlen Reading Strategies Questionnaire (free online at www.irlen.com). Students who score high on this assessment are then screened for the appropriate colored overlay by the staff member who has become an Irlen screener (Certification as an Irlen screener is a relatively inexpensive two-day process.)

b. A standard vocabulary and reading level pre- and post-program assessment should be done to identify the students' reading grade levels. I have used the Nelson-Denny reading level assessment for my college and adult students and the grade-appropriate Gates-MacGinitie reading test for my middle-school-age pilot study students. There are a number of other reading-level assessment instruments that educators are familiar with and might use (note that most of these assessment instruments can be scantron-scored).

c. For assessing problems with attention, the Amen Clinic has a free online assessment for ADD and for the six ADHD subtypes that Dr. Daniel Amen has identified (www.amenclinic.com). Because ADHD is considered a psychiatric disorder, instructors in any institution will have to consider carefully whether they wish to officially assess for this problem. Consent forms will have to be modified to avoid legal, bureaucratic, and funding complications should an institution proceed with this assessment. Because attention problems can stem from many sources, and labeling students with a "disorder" or "disability" is often counterproductive, caution here is advised. Some schools use the short "Vanderbilt ADHD Diagnostic Parent (or Teacher) Rating Scale," which can be downloaded free from the Internet (www. schoolpsychiatry.org). Again, schools will need to proceed with caution and obtain parent cooperation when assessing students for ADHD.

Instructors may want to carefully detail to parents and to older students the many causes of attention problems, such as other cognitive-processing problems (Irlen Syndrome), allergies, thyroid problems, and various medical problems. After explaining the many causes of attention problems, both known and as yet undiscovered, instructors may find it advisable to have parents or older students take charge of completing the Amen ADHD assessment on their own at home.

Instructors also need to reassure parents and students that having a learning problem like dyslexia and / or ADHD does not mean that students are unintelligent and/or cannot learn. Unfortunately, too many parents and students, and even some teachers, hold this belief—which can rapidly morph into a self-fulfilling prophesy. Labeling students as "learning disabled" can be most counterproductive!

d. WordSmart has a free online vocabulary-level assessment ("Take the WordSmart Challenge" at www.wordsmart.com). In addition, WordSmart school and home programs have quite accurate assessments built into their vocabulary-building software programs. Students take these assessments before beginning the exercises and are placed by WordSmart into the appropriate volume and word group level when they begin the program. Parents and educators who wish to experience—or have their children and students experience—WordSmart's software exercises, can access free demos at www.wordsmartedu.com.

Step 4. Modify Basic Program to fit needs of institution: The Basic Program can be modified to fit the needs of the institution. The recommended software exercise times can vary from 45 minutes to one hour per day, three to five days per week, for from five to ten weeks. More is always better than less; however, younger children will do better with 45 minutes for four days per week.

A sample five-day-per-week program is presented as follows:

Monday	Tuesday	Wednesday	Thursday	Friday
Parrot Software: Visual *OR* Auditory Memory Span—*10 minutes* WordSmart Vocabulary Building *30-40 minutes**	Parrot Software: Word Memory & Discrimination —*10 minutes* WordSmart Vocabulary Building *30-40 minutes**	Parrot Software: Visual *OR* Auditory Memory Span—*10 minutes* WordSmart Vocabulary Building *30-40 minutes**	Parrot Software: Word Memory & Discrimination —*10 minutes* WordSmart Vocabulary Building *30-40 minutes**	Parrot Software: Visual *OR* Auditory Memory Span—*10 minutes* WordSmart Vocabulary Building *30-40 minutes**

*Depending on whether session is 45 or 60 minutes long

On *Mondays, Wednesdays, and Fridays,* students do ten minutes of either Visual OR Auditory Memory Span (Parrot Software), depending upon their specific learning modality weakness. Parrot Software programs track all students' progress so students can see concrete evidence of their progress, an essential factor in motivating students to continue doing the exercises. In my experience, students begin to sense their brain's increased cognitive-processing abilities as they continue the program. This sense of growing competence accompanies all of the Basic Program's exercises. These improvements in cognition bring about, in turn, increased student confidence and self-esteem, especially as students begin to notice their increased ability to successfully tackle classroom assignments. Students can increase the programs' level of difficulty as their working-memory proficiency increases.

On *Tuesdays and Thursdays*, students do ten minutes of Word Memory and Discrimination (Parrot Software), starting with the positive question exercises. Students' progress is tracked by the program and students can increase the level of difficulty as their proficiency increases.

Every day students do 30-40 minutes (depending on whether the sessions are 45 or 60 minutes long) of WordSmart's vocabulary-building software using the following exercises:

(1) Flash cards

(2) Multiple choice

(3) Column matching

(4) Sentence completion

(5) Laser review game.

Flash cards can be omitted when students appear to have a beginning grasp of the word groups they are learning. Flash cards should be assigned to students who are struggling with English or with a given word group. WordSmart's exercises are arranged in volumes, starting with the easiest words (upper-level third grade or fourth grade); each volume contains 10 to 12 groups of 20 words each.

The WordSmart Program will automatically move the student up to the next level if the student scores between 70 percent and 90 percent correct, depending on the specific exercise. Periodically, WordSmart retests the student before moving the student to a higher level. Should the student not have retained a high enough proficiency in previous levels of vocabulary understanding, then WordSmart automatically moves the student back to their present level of proficiency. In this way, long-term memory storage of vocabulary is assured. WordSmart tracks each student's progress so both students and their teachers can see concrete evidence that their efforts are improving their word knowledge.

See Appendixes B^1—B^5 for more student ability profiles and sample exercise programs.

Step 5. Reassess students at end of program: To determine students' progress at the end of the program, students are reassessed with the appropriate age- or grade-level reading instrument.

Setting up a pilot study

If an institution wants to run a pilot study to test the Basic Program's effectiveness, then at-risk students should be assigned at random to an experimental group (receiving the program's interventions) and to a control group. Both groups must take the appropriate pre- and post-program assessments for reading grade levels. *It is important that the experimental group students who are provided with Irlen colored overlays use these overlays for all of their reading and computing activities.* Note that not all at-risk students in a pilot study will need the Irlen transparencies. However, to ascertain the degree to which the Irlen Syndrome intervention raises students' reading levels over and above the computer exercises for memory, attention, and vocabulary problems, some of the pilot study students identified for Irlen Syndrome could have their transparencies provided at the end of the study. If the pilot study reveals, as anticipated, greater reading level gains for the students provided with the transparencies, then it would be unethical not to provide all students who need them with the transparencies.

> *The Basic Program should significantly raise students' reading levels, usually by at least one grade level. As mentioned, my college pilot study students gained, on average, nearly four grade levels with, on average, 25 hours of exercises over eight weeks—a truly phenomenal gain!*

Advantages of the Basic Program over other approaches

Many educational programs have come and gone over the past few decades. Educators who have taught for a few years have been exposed to so many programs touted to solve students' learning problems that I cannot blame any of them for skepticism regarding a new program's effectiveness. Nor do I assert that this book's Basic Program is a panacea for all student learning difficulties. No one program can possibly solve all the complex, brain-based barriers to learning that individual students manifest.

What I do know, however, is that most leading educators are unaware of the high percentage of American students who harbor one or more of these hidden barriers to reading and learning. The Spring 2005 issue of the *American Educator* is entirely devoted to the topic of "Getting it right: What needs fixing [in] standards-based reform and accountability." In a thought-provoking article, Richard F. Elmore, a leading Harvard Graduate School of Education educator, admits that educators need "to get help in diagnosing the next set of problems" (once they have succeeded in increasing student performance), and to get help from those "who know what they don't know." (Elmore, 2005, p. 47). Although this article is well and thoughtfully reasoned, it makes no specific mention of the critically important, often "invisible," barriers to student learning that this book's Basic Program addresses.

My own years of research, my pilot study learning programs, and my work with hundreds of students have taught me some of what educators don't know. The Basic Program's emphasis is on identifying and remediating the visual-perceptual and auditory processing, attention, memory, and vocabulary problems that have remained hidden from many educators and from so many students of all ages. These are the problems that need to be recognized, identified in individual students, and remediated with the effective interventions that are now available.

Brain researchers are just beginning to understand some of the many causes for dyslexia and other brain-based learning problems. Experts in brain imaging, like neuropsychiatrist Dr. Daniel Amen, are beginning to discover the many reasons for and types of attention deficits. Although Helen Irlen has worked for decades to provide help to students with visual-perceptual processing problems, only in recent years have her discoveries been validated by university and U.S. Navy research studies.

Although our knowledge of learning problems is still quite incomplete, there are some solid facts upon which we can all agree:

First, American literacy levels are too low, and too many American students of all ages struggle to read with proficiency.

Second, the number of students with learning problems and below-grade-level reading ability is unacceptably high.

Third, new research in the brain sciences has revealed that the human brain— throughout the life span—is remarkably able to learn and change.

Fourth, preliminary studies support the idea that appropriate interventions and computer software exercises can "rewire" students' brains and strengthen the abilities that they need to help them read and learn to their full potential.

The United States Department of Education has established a Department of Educational Sciences whose "Cognition and Student Learning Grants" are designed to encourage researchers and educators to bring the latest breakthroughs from cognitive neuroscience laboratories into the classroom (Lyon, 1998). As a result, there has been an explosion of books and software programs claiming to do just that. A few years ago, Scientific Learning's website reported that looking for links using the words "brain" and "education" generated more than 400,000 relevant sites. When I put these two words into a Google search recently, I was presented with over 81,100,000 sites! The pertinent question now is, how can educators possibly know which of all these programs presently available are the most effective? The obvious answer is that, at this early stage, educators cannot know.

However, as an educator who has been on a decades-long search for answers to students' learning problems, I am confident that I have identified the central and overlapping problems that high percentages of American students struggle to overcome. In addition, I have found and tested programs and interventions that are effective in removing those learning barriers critically important to American students' academic success. As I have documented, the scientific evidence that supports the effectiveness of *A Practical Guide*'s programs is compelling. For example, the Irlen Syndrome has research evidence from Harvard Medical school, the University of Utah, and from the U.S. Navy, as well as from many universities in England and Australia that links this visual-perceptual processing problem to the eye's receptor fields and to the brain's magnocellular systems. Magnocellular systems in the auditory cortex are also implicated as causing some of the most common forms of auditory-processing dyslexia. In visual-perceptual and auditory-processing areas of dyslexics' brains, these magnocells appear unable to process visual and auditory stimuli rapidly enough for fluent reading (Chase, 2005; Harvard Medical School, 1994; Irvine, 2005; Livingstone et al., 1991; Tallal, 1993).

As the causes for problems are located in the brain, educational systems are becoming more receptive to adopting interventions for these problems. Ironically, some interventions have been available for many decades, including Helen Irlen's colored overlays. In March of 2004, the Massachusetts' Commissioner of Education sent out an Internet "Update" addressed to "Superintendents and Leaders of Charter Schools and Collaboratives," informing these educators about Irlen Syndrome screening as an "innovative program" promising to help the state's many struggling readers (Driscoll, 2004). Books about dyslexia and ADD are growing in number, as are books and programs designed to be "brain-based." (Wolfe, 2001).

This book's Basic Program is grounded in the now solid, evidence-based knowledge that many struggling readers and learners have remediable brain-based problems. The exact number of students nationally who could be significantly helped by the Basic Program is not knowable at this time, given the "invisible" nature of many students' learning problems, and given that many educators are unaware of how widespread these problems are in American student populations. However, given that some degree of attention deficit affects more students than any other "disorder" and appears to be a growing phenomenon, given that researchers like Dr. Sally Shaywitz are finding as many as one in five children affected by dyslexia, given that Irlen Syndrome appears to be a widespread barrier to fluency in reading, given that the number of students identified as "learning disabled" is growing and that the number of students requiring remedial or developmental classes is huge, given all of these factors, the need for a program like *A Practical Guide's* Basic Program is compelling.

Rationale for the Basic Program

The Basic Program identifies the most common learning barriers that students harbor, namely, problems in their visual and auditory systems, their memory and attention systems, and their vocabulary abilities. Taken together, I believe that identifying and remediating problems in these systems and skills will significantly help at least half of American students of all ages.

Will the Basic Program solve *all* of the learning difficulties of American students? Certainly not. There will be many students whose difficulties do not readily lend themselves to the Basic Program's remediations. Will the Basic Program solve *many* of the learning difficulties of American students? Yes, indeed, because most learning difficulties are caused by the problems I have discussed. Additionally, many students' learning problems find their sources in poor nutrition, English as a second language, and poverty. I am certain that these students, too, will be helped by the Basic Program's remediations. However, until these serious problems—especially the critical problem of poverty—are addressed effectively, many students will continue to fall behind in reading and fail to learn enough to function as productive citizens in twenty-first century America. We Americans who are interested in competing successfully in the twenty-first century's global village have much work ahead of us.

Although this book's Basic Program can't solve every student's learning difficulties, I do think that as pilot study data and cognitive neuroscience research findings continue to accumulate, the evidence will show that the Basic Program can do much to support success in learning for large numbers of American students of all ages.

Suggested Reading

Bender, W. N. (1997). *Understanding ADHD: A practical guide for teachers and parents.* Upper Saddle River, NJ: Prentice-Hall.

Goleman, D. (1995). *Emotional intelligence: Why it can matter more than IQ.* New York: Bantam Books.

Goleman, D. (2006). *Social intelligence: The new science of human relationships.* New York: Bantam Books.

Gopnik, A., Meltzoff, A. N., & Kuhl, P. K. (2001). *The scientist in the crib: What early learning tells us about the mind.* New York: HarperCollins.

Gottman, J. (1998). *Raising an emotionally intelligent child: The heart of parenting.* New York: Simon & Schuster.

Johnson, L.A. (2005). *Teaching outside the box: How to grab your students by their brains.* San Francisco: Jossey-Bass.

Quartz, S. R., & Sejnowski, T. J. (2003). *Liars, lovers, and heroes: What the new brain science reveals about how we become who we are.* New York: Quill.

Sternberg, R. J. (2001). *Successful intelligence: How practical and creative intelligence determine success in life.* New York: Simon & Schuster.

Wolfe, P. (2001). *Brain matters: Translating research into classroom practice.* Alexandria, VA: Association for Supervision and Curriculum Development.

Zentall, S. S. (2006). *ADHD and education: Foundations, characteristics, methods, and collaboration.* Upper Saddle River, N. J.: Pearson Education.

CHAPTER FIVE

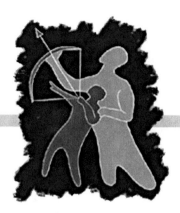

Conclusion
Using the Basic Program to create eager learners

Significant improvement in reading and learning abilities will reward those students who have used *A Practical Guide*'s Basic Program to identify their reading and learning barriers and who also have done the corresponding remediation exercises for 24 hours over six weeks. Sample ability profiles, along with the corresponding sample remediation exercises, are presented in Appendixes B^1-B^5. Parents can fill in the ability profile in Appendixes A or B^5 that best fits their children's identified learning barriers and then set up a remediation program for their children by examining the remediation exercises that correspond to the barriers identified. Older students can take the assessments provided, identify their learning barriers and, by examining the sample ability profiles, they can use the sample programs to set up their individualized remediation program.

After completing the 24 hours of remediation, students will have gained confidence in their ability to improve academically, and they will have greater insight into how they can become accomplished learners. As students' confidence and self-esteem increase, students' test anxiety will decrease. My pilot studies with students from middle-school age to adult demonstrated that as students' vocabulary, memory, and attention abilities improved, so, too, did their motivation to continue learning. Because the software exercise programs track student improvement, students will see the objective results of their efforts on the program graphs at the end of each exercise session. Subjectively, students may not have the words to express what they are experiencing but, as one of my students exclaimed, they will feel that their "synapses are really firing well!" I have seen many discouraged learners become enthusiastic learners while working on this book's Basic Program.

Brain and body health for life-long learning success

Interacting with the ongoing revolution in knowledge about learning and the brain is a revolution in our understanding of mental and physical health problems. Americans have become aware of an obesity epidemic among the young that is troubling because children who are overweight tend not to be able to perform either physically or intellectually to their full potential. At the same time, Americans have also become aware of the growing numbers of students identified with so-called learning "disabilities" like ADHD and visual-perceptual and auditory-processing dyslexias. I think that these two societal problems are closely related.

First, American children, like their elders, are bombarded daily with toxic stress in the form of competitive academic, sport, and social challenges. Toxic stress also comes, I would argue, in the form of leisure activities that involve destructive and violent video games and television programs. Some years ago, New York Senator Daniel Patrick Moynihan decried what he called the "coarsening of the culture." Children who are continuously exposed to violent images of warfare—real and fictional—are in danger of a desensitization that robs them of their humanity. Medical researchers are beginning to understand the relationship between a competitive, violent, and stressful environment and obesity. Of course, the typical American lifestyle—fast food, little or no exercise, and lack of sufficient sleep—is also implicated in the American obesity epidemic.

When students' attention is constantly deflected at short intervals by the loud, fast, and nerve-jangling sounds and images of news, commercials, and entertainment, an inability to focus and pay attention for long periods is programmed into their nervous systems. When students' minds and bodies are not provided with nourishing sleep, or with the essential nutrients their brains require to function optimally, students cannot concentrate on challenging information and learn to think critically. Most Americans are not undernourished; but we Americans are certainly malnourished—we don't eat the right food! The obesity outbreak among American children is leading to epidemics of diseases that can conceivably doom American children's brain power—even before they reach adulthood.

Parents concerned about their children's academic success are also concerned about their children's mind and brain health. Children, as well as adults, who do not get adequate sleep are more apt to become overweight. Exercise, good nutrition, and adequate sleep have a profound effect on memory and learning. Moreover, the American fast-food diet is lacking in the essential fatty acids, particularly the omega-3s, which support brain / mind systems. The brain is at least 60 percent fat, mostly omega-3s, and these omega-3 fatty acids not only support optimal brain function, but they also are essential for the eyes' visual pathways. The lack of omega-3 fatty acids in the typical American diet could explain why ADHD and Irlen Syndrome visual-perceptual dyslexia appear to be increasing problems for American youth (Sears, 2005, 2002; Stordy & Nicholl, 2000).

Researchers at Purdue University, as well as at universities in England, have found significant benefit for children with a variety of learning problems ranging from ADHD to dyslexia, to the "clumsy child" syndrome (dyspraxia), when supplementation with purified fish oil capsules is provided. These fish oil capsules contain the omega-3 fatty acids essential for optimum brain development (Stevens, 2000; Stordy & Nicholl, 2000).

Earlier generations of children in America and Europe were given cod liver oil, which was understood to promote optimum brain development. When I ask my adult students if they were given cod liver oil as children, a few students in their forties or fifties will make a face expressing disgust and signal that, yes, they remember swallowing the awful stuff. Now, of course, besides the repugnant taste of cod liver oil, there is the valid concern about the heavy metals and other pollutants that contaminate fish and fish oils. Parents wishing to support their children's brain development would do well to read books like Stordy and Nicholl's *The LCP [long-chain polyunsaturated fatty acid] Solution: The remarkable nutritional treatment for ADHD, dyslexia, & dyspraxia*. Parents could also visit neuropsychiatrist Dr. Daniel Amen's website (www.amenclinics. com) and read archived editions of his *Brain in the News* articles on "Fish Oil and Coordination" and "Fish Protect the Brain." In addition, Dr. Amen has archived "Supplements to Enhance the Brain: A Summary of Ways to Optimize Brain Function and Break Bad Brain Habits."

Parents are beginning to demand natural treatments to help their children who are experiencing problems with hyperactivity, concentration, memory, and dyslexia. With recent research findings that indicate many dangerous side effects for some of the standard medications for ADHD (Ritalin for example) parents are wise to investigate fish oil supplementation, or other natural substances like vitamins, herbs, and amino acids to support their children's optimum brain functioning (Bryan et al., 2004). As the father of three children with ADD, Dr. Amen is especially interested in treatments that can help his patients of all ages overcome their learning problems. Dr. Amen, however, does warn that parents should always consult with their children's doctors before giving them *any* supplements, especially if the children are already taking medications. Furthermore, because the diet or supplements that may help one type of ADD may not be helpful for another type of ADD, parents would be wise to visit Dr. Amen's website and investigate Dr. Amen's free Brain Systems tests to identify, first, if their children have ADD and, second, the type of ADD their children appear to have. Dr. Amen's free recommendations for diet, supplementation, and medication are different for each ADD subtype.

Is America an "ADDogenic" culture?

Some experts in the field of attention deficits have remarked that our culture elicits a degree of attention deficit behavior from us all (Hallowell & Ratey, 1994). In brief, Americans are living in a society of sleep-deprived and malnourished individuals who are addicted to junk food, TV, and video games! The obesity epidemic reflects our American "over" nutrition that, nonetheless, represents malnourishment. Many Americans are damaging their brains—and their unborn children's brains—with even more sinister addictions to tobacco, drugs, and alcohol. Fortunately, experts in many disciplines have begun to question American society's destructive eating, sleeping, "couch-potato" habits, and stress-inducing pressures. Another fortunate development is the concern expressed by American parents who are limiting their children's exposure to violent TV and video games and programs, as well as monitoring their children's diet and exercise regimens.

In sum, there are many plausible reasons for what appears a very real increase in attention-deficit problems. Besides the genetic factors producing ADD and ADHD brains, our country's problems with addictive behaviors—of both mother and father—are producing more brain-damaged children who have learning difficulties ranging from mild to severe. Added to this mix are the nearly 20 percent of American children growing up in poverty who often are poorly nourished both physically and mentally and who are, therefore, at greater risk for problems with attention and focus. My colleagues in the elementary schools have told me that we college instructors will be teaching in the near future increasing numbers of students with ADHD. I think that this "future" is now.

Therefore, I am urging all readers of this short program book to educate themselves about the brain's need for the essential nutrients lacking in the typical American diet, and to become informed about the need everyone has for adequate sleep and moderate daily exercise to ensure optimal mental, physical, and emotional health. We Americans would do well to heed the ancient Greek motto, "A healthy mind in a healthy body."

Finally, the latest news from the brain sciences emphasizes the "use-it-or-lose-it" principle in regard to mental acuity. Our rapidly changing global marketplace mandates that we all become life-long learners continuously upgrading our marketable skills. A welcome consequence of these pressures, once we learn to live with them in a balanced way, ensures that we will continue to exercise our minds and brains, just as we exercise our bodies. For example, studies of individuals who avoid succumbing to Alzheimer's disease, even in late old age, reveal that these are the individuals who have remained mentally active and engaged in life—all their lives. Medical researchers now believe that even individuals with a genetic heritage that makes them susceptible to Alzheimer's can delay its onset with continued mental activity, perhaps even long enough to avoid the significant mental decline that is this terrible disease's hallmark.

Therefore, in conclusion, I hope that parents and their children will use this book's Basic Program to identify and decrease, or even eliminate, those invisible barriers to reading and learning that are keeping them from academic and professional success. I also hope that by finally experiencing this success, parents and their children will be inspired to learn more about the role that a healthy lifestyle and continuing mental activity can play in their future success as life-long learners.

Suggested reading

Amen, D. G., M. D. (2005). *Making a good brain great.* New York: Random House.

Sears, B. (2005). *The anti-inflammation zone: Reversing the silent epidemic that's destroying our health.* New York: Harper Collins.

Sears, B. (2002). *The omega Rx zone: The miracle of the new high-dose fish oil.* New York: HarperCollins.

Stevens, L. (2000). *12 effective ways to help your ADD / ADHD child.* New York: Avery.

Stordy, B. J., & Nicholl, M. J. (2000). *The LCP solution: The remarkable nutritional treatment for ADHD, dyslexia& dyspraxia.* New York: Ballantine.

Weil, A., M. D. (2000). *Eating well for optimum health: The essential guide to food, diet, and nutrition.* New York: Alfred A. Knopf.

Appendix A

Key Student Abilities Profile

First: Using the student ability assessments gained from the WordSmart vocabulary assessment, the Parrot Software questionnaire (memory and attention), and the Amen Clinic's "Brain Systems" assessment for attention, parents and older students can fill in their individual ability profile [IAP] on the bar graph provided above.

Second: By examining the sample remediation exercises presented in Appendixes B[1], B[2], B[3], and B[4], parents and older students can design an individual remediation program [IRP] that can raise the abilities critical for enhanced reading and learning.

Appendix B[1]

A sample remediation program for students whose main learning difficulty is low memory

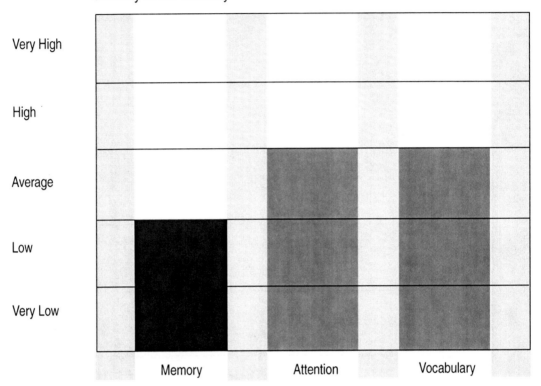

The Basic Program requires that students with low memory ability do remediation exercises at least four times a week for one hour using the following exercises:

Parrot Software: Use "Visual and Auditory Memory Span" for 15 minutes a day, alternating auditory and visual modes and increasing the number of letters or numbers as proficiency is gained.

Use "Word Memory and Discrimination" for 15 minutes a day, alternating between modalities and category inclusion / exclusion until proficiency is reached.

WordSmart: Use the vocabulary-building exercises in the order provided for 30 minutes per day at the appropriate volume and word-group level. *Note* that WordSmart assesses each student's vocabulary level, places the student in the appropriate volume and word group, and tracks each student's progress. WordSmart will move the student to the next level as word proficiency is gained.

Appendix B[2]

A sample remediation program for students whose main learning difficulty is low attention

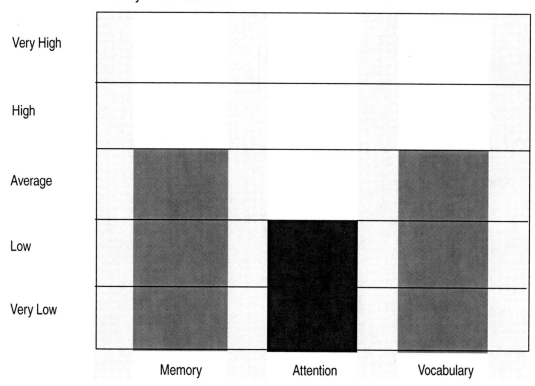

The Basic Program requires that students with low attention ability do remediation exercises at least four times a week for one hour using the following exercises:

Parrot Software: Use "Hierarchical Attention Training" for 20 minutes a day, alternating attention conditions and slowly increasing difficulty levels as proficiency is reached.

Use "Visual and Auditory Memory Span" for 10 minutes a day, alternating auditory and visual modes and increasing the number of letters or numbers as proficiency is gained.

WordSmart: Use the vocabulary-building exercises in the order provided for 30 minutes per day at the appropriate volume and word-group level. *Note* that WordSmart assesses each student's vocabulary level, places the student in the appropriate volume and word group, and tracks each student's progress. WordSmart will move the student to the next level as word proficiency is gained.

Appendix B[3]

A sample remediation program for students with low vocabulary ability.

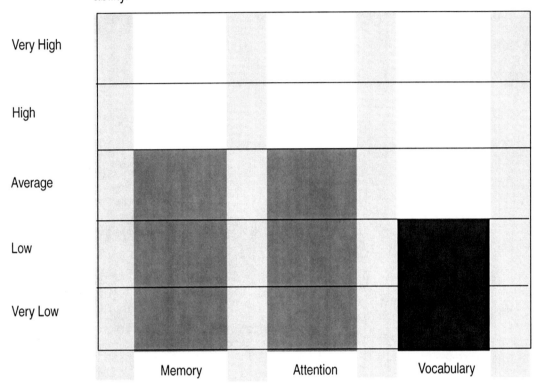

The Basic Program requires that students with low vocabulary ability do remediation exercises at least four times a week for one hour using the following exercises:

Parrot Software: Use "Visual and Auditory Memory Span" for 15 minutes a day, alternating auditory and visual modes and increasing the number of letters or numbers as proficiency is gained.

WordSmart: Use the vocabulary-building exercises in the order provided for 45 minutes per day at the appropriate volume and word-group level. *Note* that WordSmart assesses each student's vocabulary level, places the student in the appropriate volume and word group, and tracks each student's progress. WordSmart will move the student to the next level as word proficiency is gained.

Appendix B⁴

A sample remediation program for students who have three learning difficulty areas.

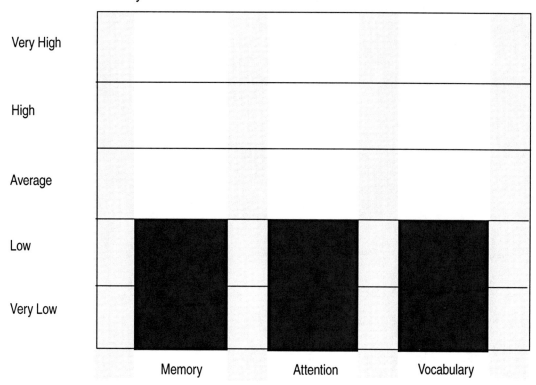

The Basic Program requires that students with three low ability areas do remediation exercises at least four times a week for one hour using the following exercises: (These students may need to continue the Basic Program longer than students with only one or two low ability areas.)

Parrot Software: Use "Hierarchical Attention Training" for 15 minutes a day, alternating attention conditions and slowly increasing difficulty levels as proficiency is reached.

Use "Visual and Auditory Memory Span" for 15 minutes a day, alternating auditory and visual modes and increasing the number of letters or numbers as proficiency is gained.

WordSmart: Use the vocabulary-building exercises in the order provided for 30 minutes per day at the appropriate volume and word-group level. NOTE that WordSmart assesses each student's vocabulary level, places the student in the appropriate volume and word group, and tracks each student's progress. WordSmart will move the student to the next level as word proficiency is gained.

Appendix B[5]

A sample program for preschool and early elementary students that can help remediate and prevent reading and learning difficulties (parents can color in estimated ability levels below and vary the times and programs accordingly.

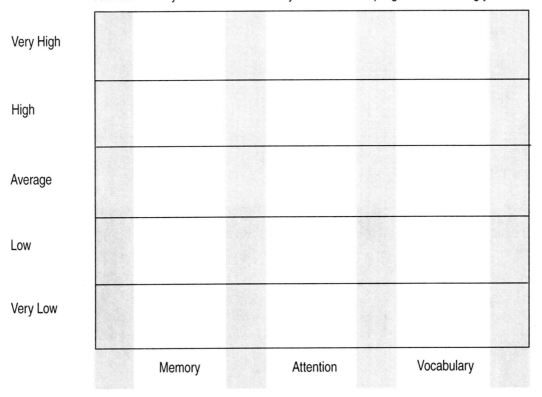

The Basic Program for preschool and early elementary students may remediate, as well as prevent, reading and learning difficulties. The Basic Program requires that these young students do the following exercises three or four times a week for 40—50 minutes.

Parrot Software: Use two programs a day, alternating among the following four programs:

- Use "Visual Memory" for ten minutes on alternate days.
- Use "Listening Skills" for ten minutes on alternate days.
- Use "Visual and Auditory Memory Span" for ten minutes on alternate days.
- Use "Attention Perception and Discrimination" for ten minutes (older students) on alternate days.

WordSmart: Use WordSmart's phonics program for 15 to 20 minutes per day, depending upon the student's age and developmental level. Older students may want to continue for 30 minutes.

Appendix C
Reading Enhancement & Computerized Learning
The Basic Program Student Schedule

The Basic Program requires one hour of practice per day (40 to 50 minutes per day for younger students), four days a week (students can do more if they wish) for five to six weeks. Students with multiple barriers to learning will need to extend the Basic Program for additional weeks. (A preprogram reading level assessment and a post-program reading level assessment is desirable for institutional tracking of student progress.)

Parents and students may keep track of practice dates and times on the following agenda:

Week One

Date:_____Time: *WordSmart:* _____ Time: *Parrot Software:* _____

Date: _____Time: *WordSmart:* _____ Time: *Parrot Software:* _____

Date: _____Time: *WordSmart:* _____ Time: *Parrot Software:* _____

Date: _____Time: *WordSmart:* _____ Time: *Parrot Software:* _____

Date: _____Time: *WordSmart:* _____ Time: *Parrot Software:* _____

Week Two

Date:_____Time: *WordSmart:* _____ Time: *Parrot Software:* _____

Date: _____Time: *WordSmart:* _____ Time: *Parrot Software:* _____

Date: _____ Time: *WordSmart:* _____ Time: *Parrot Software:* _____

Date: _____Time: *WordSmart:* _____ Time: *Parrot Software:* _____

Date: _____Time: *WordSmart:* _____ Time: *Parrot Software:* _____

Continued on the following page

Week Three

Date:_____Time: *WordSmart:* _____ Time: *Parrot Software:* _____

Date:_____Time: *WordSmart:* _____ Time: *Parrot Software:* _____

Date:_____Time: *WordSmart:* _____ Time: *Parrot Software:* _____

Date:_____Time: *WordSmart:* _____ Time: *Parrot Software:* _____

Date:_____Time: *WordSmart:* _____ Time: *Parrot Software:* _____

Week Four

Date:_____Time: *WordSmart:* _____ Time: *Parrot Software:* _____

Date:_____Time: *WordSmart:* _____ Time: *Parrot Software:* _____

Date:_____Time: *WordSmart:* _____ Time: *Parrot Software:* _____

Date:_____Time: *WordSmart:* _____ Time: *Parrot Software:* _____

Date:_____Time: *WordSmart:* _____ Time: *Parrot Software:* _____

Week Five

Date:_____Time: *WordSmart:* _____ Time: *Parrot Software:* _____

Date:_____Time: *WordSmart:* _____ Time: *Parrot Software:* _____

Date:_____Time: *WordSmart:* _____ Time: *Parrot Software:* _____

Date:_____Time: *WordSmart:* _____ Time: *Parrot Software:* _____

Date:_____Time: *WordSmart:* _____ Time: *Parrot Software:* _____

Week Six

Date:_____Time: *WordSmart:* _____ Time: *Parrot Software:* _____

Date:_____Time: *WordSmart:* _____ Time: *Parrot Software:* _____

Date:_____Time: *WordSmart:* _____ Time: *Parrot Software:* _____

Date:_____Time: *WordSmart:* _____ Time: *Parrot Software:* _____

Date:_____Time: *WordSmart:* _____ Time: *Parrot Software:* _____

Appendix D

The Basic Program's Sample Institutional Consent Form
(Institution's name here) Parental Consent Form

Reading Enhancement and Computerized Skill-Building Educational Program

Purposes & Benefits

Dear Parents:

Your child has the opportunity to participate in a reading and learning program that has the potential to significantly improve your child's reading and learning abilities. Your child will be screened for reading difficulties that may be caused by light sensitivity, a reading difficulty recognized by several states' educational districts.

An Irlen "Reading Strategies Questionnaire" will be given to your child, along with a Grade Level Reading Assessment. Depending upon the results of these two educational assessments, your child will be provided with help for light sensitivity (colored transparencies to place over the computer screen and over reading materials), along with 24 hours over six weeks of computerized enrichment exercises that are evidence-based and designed to enhance your child's reading and learning abilities.

The Reading Enhancement and Computerized Skill-Building Exercises can improve your child's auditory and visual working memory, attention / focus, and vocabulary skills.

Procedures

The Reading Strategies Questionnaire takes about 10 minutes to complete; the Grade Level Reading Assessment requires just under an hour to administer. Your child will be asked to complete these assessments before the enrichment program begins. Your child will be asked to complete a post-program Grade Level Reading Assessment after the enrichment program has ended to provide grade level improvement data.

Risks, Stress & Discomfort

If any information related to this program is released, individual subjects will not be identified. Data from this study will be used for educational research to improve students' reading/ learning abilities, and to help improve students' performance on your state's assessment of student learning tests. There should be no substantial stress or discomfort involved. Your child may withdraw from this program at any time. There are no guarantees as to improvement in your child's reading/learning abilities, but based on previous pilot study data, and on research supporting this approach, your child should benefit from participation in this program. If your child does decide to withdraw from the program before its conclusion, then improvement data will not be available to you or to your child.

_____

Signature of Pilot Study Director   Date

_____

Signature of School Administrator   Date

Subject Parents' Statement:

This reading/learning program described above has been explained to me, and I and my child have had an opportunity to ask questions. I understand that future questions I may have about this program will be answered by the Pilot Study Director named above or by the Director of the school enrichment program.

I hereby give permission for my child to participate in this Reading Enhancement and Computerized Learning Program.

PLEASE SIGN AND DATE:

_____

Signature of Mother   Date

PLEASE PRINT YOUR NAME:_____

Telephone number where you can be reached:

Daytime:_____ Evening: _____

_____

Signature of Father   Date

PLEASE PRINT YOUR NAME:_____

Telephone number where you can be reached:

Daytime: _____ Evening: _____

_____

Signature of Student   Date

PLEASE PRINT YOUR NAME: _____

Appendix E

The Basic Program's Institutional Implementation Plan

Note that this Reading Enhancement and Computerized Learning Program has been developed over the past decade and has served hundreds of students ranging in age from ten to fifty years old. With the Irlen Syndrome intervention, as needed, and 24 hours, on average, of computerized remediation for memory, attention, and vocabulary, pilot study students have gained a minimum of one year in reading grade level. Most students have gained several years of reading grade level, with some demonstrating gains of up to five years. Pilot study students have reported improvements in their test-taking abilities and grades.

Steps for Basic Program implementation:

First: Institutional consent forms are signed by participating parents and students.

Second: Students are given a reading grade-level assessment test.

Third: Students are assessed for Irlen Syndrome, a type of visual-perceptual dyslexia prevalent among struggling students. Irlen Syndrome is easy to remediate: The remediation consists of colored transparencies placed over reading materials and over computer screens. This effective intervention is permitted on many school districts' state standards tests.

Fourth: Students are provided with appropriately-colored transparencies for Irlen Syndrome, if needed.

Fifth: Students are assigned four hours per week, for six weeks, of computerized software exercises to improve their attention and working-memory abilities, and to raise their vocabulary levels.

Sixth: Students are reassessed for their reading grade level after they have completed 24 hours of ability-raising computer exercises.

Institutions may decide to continue the Basic Program for longer periods to achieve even greater reading and learning ability improvements.

Please note that all of the components of this Reading Enhancement and Computerized Learning Program are evidence based.

Selected References

Adler, J. (1999, June 28). Stress isn't just a catchall complaint: It's being linked to heart disease, immune deficiency and memory loss. *Newsweek (International Ed.), 133*, 48-53.

Allen, L. R., & Sethi, A. (Summer, 2004). Bridging the gap between poor and privileged: How the parent-child home program uses books and toys to help poor toddlers succeed in kindergarten and beyond. *American Educator, 28*, 34-42, 54-55.

Alpert, R., & Nader, R. N. (1960). *Instruments for adults: Achievement anxiety test (AAT)*. American Psychological Association.

Amen, D. G., M.D. (1998). *Change your brain, change your life: The breakthrough program for conquering anxiety, depression, obsessiveness, anger, and impulsiveness*. New York: Times Books.

Amen, D. G., M. D. (2005). *Making a good brain great*. New York: Harmony Books.

Amen, D. G., M. D. (2005). *Making a good brain great*. Presentation at the Irlen International Institute's North American Conference, July 22, 2005.

Andreano, J. M., & Cahill, L. (2006). Research report: Glucocorticoid release and memory consolidation in men and women. *Psychological Science, 17*, 466.

Ashcraft, M. H., & Kirk, E. P. (2001). The relationships among working memory, math anxiety, and performance. *Journal of Experimental Psychology: General, 130*, 224-237.

Barkley, R. A. (1997). *ADHD and the nature of self-control*. New York: Guilford.

Beatty, J. (2001). *The human brain: Essentials of behavioral neuroscience*. Thousand Oaks, CA.: Sage Publications, Inc.

Begley, S. (1996). The IQ puzzle: Scores on intelligence tests around the world have risen sharply. Does the baffling increase mean that today's children are near geniuses? Or do IQ tests reveal less about intelligence than we think? *Newsweek, 127*(19), 70-72.

Bell, S. M., McCallum, R. S., & Cox, E. A. (2003). Toward a research-based assessment of dyslexia: Using cognitive measures to identify reading disabilities. *Journal of Learning Disabilities, 36*, 505-516.

Bender, W. N. (1997). *Understanding ADHD: A practical guide for teachers and parents.* Upper Saddle River, NJ: Merrill/Prentice-Hall.

Biemiller, A. (Spring, 2001). Teaching vocabulary: Early, direct, and sequential. *American Educator, 25*, 24-28.

Bowker, R. (1977). Comparison of the vocabulary knowledge of high and low verbal-SAT students. *Johnson O'Connor Research Foundation*, Human Engineering Laboratory.

Brubaker, C. L. (2005). *LD from the inside out: A survival guide for parents.* Casper, WY: Whiskey Creek Press.

Bruer, J. T. (1999). Neural connections: Some you use, some you lose. *Phi Delta Kappan, 81*, 264-277.

Bryan, J., Osendarp, S., Hughes, D., Calvaresi, E., Baghurst, K., & van Klinken, J-W. (2004). Nutrients for cognitive development in school-aged children. *Nutrition Reviews, 62*, 295-306.

Cahill, L., & McGaugh, J. L. (1998). Mechanisms of emotional arousal and lasting declarative memory. *Trends in Neurosciences, 21*, 294-300.

Catone, W. V., & Brady, S. A. (2005). The inadequacy of individual educational program (IEP) goals for high school students with word-level reading difficulties. *Annals of Dyslexia, 55*, 53-79.

Chall, J. S., & Jacobs, V. A. (Spring, 2003). Poor children's fourth grade slump. *American Educator, 27*, 14-15.

Chase, C. (2005). *Magnocellular cone signal strength and reading.* Presentation at the Irlen International Institute's North American Conference. July 22, 2005.

Chenausky, K. (1997). Training dyslexics first to hear, then to read. *MIT's Technology Review, 100,* 15-17.

Christakis, D. (2005). Television watching and shortened attention spans. *Pediatrics for Parents, 21,* 10-12.

Coles, G. (2004). Danger in the classroom: 'Brain glitch' research and learning to read, *Phi Delta Kappan, 85,* 344-353.

Cynkar, A. (March, 2007). Conversing with copycats: Psychologists are using computer models to re-evaluate how humans learn their first tongue. *Monitor on Psychology, 38,* 46.

Daniel, S. S., Walsh, A. K., Goldston, D. B., & Arnold, E. M. (2006). Suicidality, school drop out, and reading problems among adolescents. *Journal of Learning Disabilities, 39,* 507-515.

Davis, R. D., with Braun, E. M. (1997). *The gift of dyslexia: Why some of the smartest people can't read and how they can learn.* New York: Perigee.

Demonet, J-F., Taylor, M. J., & Chaix, Y. (2004). Developmental dyslexia. *The Lancet, 363,* 1451-61.

Dingfelder, S. F. (February, 2007). Your brain on video games. *Monitor on Psychology, 20,* 21.

Driscoll, D. P. (March 22, 2004). *Commissioner's update: A new tool to help improve reading scores. Irlen / Scotopic Sensitivity Syndrome.* Massachusetts Department of Education. Downloaded 3/24/2004: http://www.doe.mass.edu/mailings/2004/cm032204.html.

Elmore, R. F. (Spring, 2005). Building new knowledge: School improvement requires new knowledge, not just good will. *American Educator, 29,* 20-27, 47.

Eisner, E. W. (2004). Multiple intelligences: Its tensions and possibilities. *Teachers College Record, 106,* 31-39.

Evans, G. W. (2004). The environment of childhood poverty. *American Psychologist, 59,* 77-92.

Gang, M., & Siegel, L. S. (2002). Sound-symbol learning in children with dyslexia. *Journal of Learning Disabilities, 35,* 137-157.

Gardner, H. (1983). *Frames of mind: The theory of multiple intelligences.* New York: Basic Books.

Gillespie, K. (April 17, 2001). How vision impacts literacy: An educational problem that can be solved. *Harvard Graduate School of Education News.* www.gse.harvard.edu/news/features/vision04172001

Goleman, D. (1995). *Emotional intelligence: Why it can matter more than IQ.* New York: Bantam Books.

Goleman, D. (2006). *Social intelligence: The new science of human relationships.* New York: Bantam Books.

Gopnik, A., Meltzoff, A. N., & Kuhl, P. K. (2001). *The scientist in the crib: What early learning tells us about the mind.* New York: Perennial.

Gottman, J. (1998). *Raising an emotionally intelligent child: The heart of parenting.* New York: Fireside.

Hallowell, E. M., M.D., & Ratey, J. J., M.D. (2006). *Delivered from distraction: Getting the most out of life with attention deficit disorder.* New York: Ballantine Books.

Hallowell, E. M., M.D., & Ratey, J. J., M.D. (1995). *Driven to distraction: Recognizing and coping with attention deficit disorder from childhood through adulthood.* New York: Pantheon Books.

Hamilton, S. S., M.D., & Glasco, F. P. (2006). Evaluation of children with reading difficulties. *American Family Physician, 74,* 2079-84.

Harding, K. L., Judah, R. D., & Gant, C. E., M.D. (2003). Outcome-based comparison of Ritalin versus food-supplement treated children with AD/HD. *Alternative Medicine Review, 8,* 319-330.

Hart, B., & Risley, T. R. (Spring, 2003). The early catastrophe: The 30 million word gap by age 3. *American Educator, 27,* 4-9.

Hartnett, D. N., Nelson, J. M., & Rinn, A. N. (2004). Gifted or ADHD? The possibilities of misdiagnosis. *Roeper Review, 26,* 73-77.

Harvard Medical School. (Jan. 21, 1994). Eye spy: Decoding dyslexia. *Focus,* A Publication of Harvard Medical School.

Hecker, L., Burns, L., Elkind, J., Elkind, K., & Katz, L. (2002). Benefits of assistive reading software for students with attention disorders. *Annals of Dyslexia, 52,* 243-273.

Heiervany, E., & Hugdahl, K. (2003). Impaired visual attention in children with dyslexia, *Journal of Learning Disabilities, 36,* 68-74.

Hirsch, E.D., Jr. (Spring, 2003). Reading comprehension requires knowledge—or words and the world: Scientific insights into the fourth-grade slump and stagnant reading comprehension. *American Educator, 27,* 10-13, 16-22, 28-29, 48.

Horgan, J. (1996). Playing past learning disabilities. *Scientific American, 275,* 102.

Howes, N. L., Bigler, E. D., Burlingame, G. M., & Lawson, J. S. (2003). Memory performance of children with dyslexia: A comparative analysis of theoretical perspectives. *Journal of Learning Disabilities, 36,* 230-246.

Hudson, R. F., High, L., & Otaiba, S. A. (2007). Dyslexia and the brain: What does current research tell us? *The Reading Teacher, 60,* 506-515.

Irlen, H. (2005). (Updated Edition). *Reading by the colors: Overcoming dyslexia and other reading disabilities through the Irlen method.* New York: Perigee.

Irlen, H. L. (1994). Scotopic sensitivity / Irlen syndrome: Hypothesis and explanation of the syndrome. *Journal of Behavioral Optometry, 5,* 2-6.

Irlen, H., & Robinson, G. L. (1996). The effect of Irlen colored filters on adult perception of workplace performance: A preliminary survey. *Australian Journal of Learning Disabilities, 1,* 7-16.

Irlen, H., & Yellen, A. G. (2007). *Reducing combat stress and Irlen Syndrome.* Presentation to the 15th Annual International Civilian & Military Combat Stress Conference, May 4-10, 2007. Camp Pendleton, CA.

Irvine, J. H. (2005). *The cause of Irlen syndrome.* Presentation at Irlen International Institute's North American Conference, July 23, 2005.

Jensen, E. (2001). Fragile brains: Understanding learning differences. *Educational Leadership, 59,* 1-7.

Johnson, LA. (2005). *Teaching outside the box: How to grab your students by their brains.* San Francisco: Jossey-Bass.

Johnson, R. R., & Layng, T. V. J. (1992). Breaking the structuralist barrier: Literacy and numeracy with fluency. *American Psychologist, 47,* 1475-90.

Johnston, R. S., & Morrison, M. (2007). Towards a resolution of inconsistencies in the phonological deficit theory of reading disorders: Phonological reading difficulties are more severe in high-IQ poor readers. *Journal of Learning Disabilities, 40,* 66-80.

Kibby, M. Y., Marks, W., Morgan, S., & Long, C. J. (2004). Specific impairment in developmental reading disabilities: A working memory approach. *Journal of Learning Disabilities, 37,* 349-364.

Kleinfeld, J., & Wescott, S. (Eds.). (1993). *Fantastic Antone succeeds! Experiences in educating children with Fetal Alcohol Syndrome.* University of Alaska Press.

Kranowitz, C. S. (2005). *The out-of-sync child: Recognizing and coping with sensory processing disorder.* New York: Penguin.

Krouse, S. L., & Irvine, J. H. (2003). *Perceptual dyslexia: Its effect on the military cadre and benefits of treatment.* 45th Annual Conference of the International Military Testing Association. 3-6 November, Pensacola, FL.

Lauerman, J. F. (March, 2001). Poor reading means poor prospects. www.brainconnection. com/topics/?main=fa/47_1

Leamnson, R. (2000). Learning as biological brain change. *Change, 32,* 34-40.

Lee, J. H. (1999). Test anxiety and working memory. *Journal of Experimental Education, 67,* 218-241.

Levine, M. D., M.D. with Reed, M. R. (1999). (2nd Ed.) *Developmental variation and learning disorders.* Cambridge, MA: Educators Publishing Service, Inc.

Levine, P. (2003). *Put eye exam on back-to-school to-do list.* www.brainconnection.com.

Livingstone, M. S., Rosen, G. D., Drislane, F. W., & Galaburda, A. M. (1991). Physiological and anatomical evidence for a magnocellular defect in developmental dyslexia. *Proceedings of the National Academy of Sciences, 88,* 7943-7947.

Lubar, J. F., Swartwood, M. O., Swartwood, J. N., & O'Donnell, P. H. (1995). Evaluation of the effectiveness of EEG neurofeedback training for ADHD in a clinical setting as measured by changes in T.O.V.A. scores, behavioral ratings, and WISC-R performance. *Biofeedback and Self-Regulation, 20,* 83-99.

Lyon, G. R. (April 28, 1998). *Overview of reading and literacy initiatives.* Statement to the U.S. Senate Committee on Labor and Human Resources. www.nichd.nih.gov/crmc/cdb/r_overview

Lyytinen, P., Poikkeus, A. M., Laakso, M. L., Eklund, K. & Lyytinen, H. (2001). Language development and symbolic play in children with and without familial risk for dyslexia. *Journal of Speech, Language, and Hearing Research, 44,* 873-885.

Maloney, W. H. (2003). Connecting the texts of their lives to academic literacy: Creating success for at-risk first-year students. *Journal of Adolescent & Adult Literacy, 46,* 664-673.

Manno, B. V., & Finn, C. E. (1996). Universities in crisis: What's wrong with the American university? Behind the curtain. *The Wilson Quarterly, 20,* 44-53.

Martinez, M. E. (2000). *Education as the cultivation of intelligence.* Mahwah, NJ.: Lawrence Erlbaum Associates, Inc.

Miller, J. A. (1993). It's all in the timing. *Bioscience, 43,* 80-83.

McCrory, E. J., Mechelli, A., Frith, U., & Price, C. J. (2005). More than words: A common neural basis for reading and naming deficits in developmental dyslexia? *Brain, 128,* 261-267.

Morrow, F. (2005). *Report from the trenches: An assessment and computerized remediation program that applies cognitive neuroscience in the classroom.* Presentation at Irlen International Institute's North American Conference, July 23, 2005.

Murray, B. (2000). From brain scan to lesson plan. *Monitor on Psychology, 31,* 22-28.

Murray, B. (2003). Training young minds not to wander. *Monitor on Psychology, 34,* 58-59.

Nagarajian, S., Mahncke, H., Salz, T., Tallal, P., et al. (1999). Cortical auditory signal processing in poor readers. *Proceedings of the National Academy of Sciences of the United States of America, 96,* 6483-6488.

National Institutes of Health Consensus Statement. (1998). Rehabilitation of persons with traumatic brain injury. *National Institutes of Health, 16,* 17.

Neisser, U. (1997). Rising scores on intelligence tests. *American Scientist, 85,* 440-447.

Nelson, C. A. (1999). Neural plasticity and human development. *Current Directions in Psychological Science, 8,* 42-45.

Noble, J., Orton, M., Irlen, S., & Robinson, G. (2004). A controlled field study of the use of colored overlays on reading achievement. *Australian Journal of Learning Disabilities, 9,* 14-22.

O'Connor, P. D., Sofo, F., Kendall, L., & Olsen, G. (1990). Reading disabilities and the effects of colored filters. *Journal of Learning Disabilities, 23,* 597-603, 620.

O'Neil Bona, K., & Martin, A. (2004). The secret life of the dyslexic child: How she thinks, how he feels, how they can succeed. *The American Journal of Psychiatry, 161,* 938-940.

Parker, M. C. (2004). Photon induced visual abnormalities (PIVA) and visual dyslexia. Prepared for the *Nebraska Occupational Therapy Association Conference, 1-12,* October 9, 2004, Lincoln, NE.

Perkins, D. N. (1995). *Outsmarting IQ: The emerging science of learnable intelligence.* New York: The Free Press.

Posner, M. I. (2004). Neural systems and individual differences. *Teachers College Record, 106,* 24-31.

Posner, M. I., & Rothbart, M. K. (2005). Influencing brain networks: Implications for education. *Trends in Cognitive Sciences, 9,* 99-103.

Posner, M. I., Rothbart, M. K., & Rueda, M. R. (2003). *Brain mechanisms and learning of high level skills.* Paper presented at a meeting on Brain and Education, Papal Academy of Sciences, Vatican City.

Price, C. J., & Devlin, J. T. (2003). The myth of the visual word form area. *NeuroImage, 19,* 473-481.

Quartz, S. R., & Sejnowski, T. J. (2003). *Liars, lovers, and heroes: What the new brain science reveals about how we become who we are.* New York: Quill.

Rapin, I. (2002). Diagnostic dilemmas in developmental disabilities: Fuzzy margins at the edges of normality. An essay prompted by Thomas Sowell's new book: *The Einstein Syndrome. Journal of Autism and Developmental Disorders, 32,* 49-57.

Reiff, M. I., M.D., Banez, G. A., & Culbert, T. P., M.D. (1993). Children who have attentional disorders: Diagnosis and evaluation. *Pediatrics in Review, 14,* 455-465.

Remick, K. M., Stroud, C. A., & Bedes, V. (2000). *Eyes on track: A missing link to successful learning (Grades 1-6).* Folsom, CA: JF's Publishing.

Robbins, T. W., Mehta, M. A., & Sahakian, B. J. (2000). Boosting working memory. *Science, 290,* 2275-2276.

Robertson, I. H. (2000). *Mind sculpture: Unlocking your brain's untapped potential.* New York: Fromm International.

Robertson, I. H., & Murre, J. M. J. (1999). Rehabilitation of brain damage: Brain plasticity and principles of guided recovery. *Psychological Bulletin, 125,* 544-575.

Robinson, G. L. (1994). Colored lenses and reading: A review of research into reading achievement, reading strategies and causal mechanisms. *Australian Journal of Special Education, 18,* 3-14.

Robinson, G. L. (1997). *The familial incidence of symptoms of scotopic sensitivity / Irlen Syndrome: A more detailed analysis.* Paper presented at the Third Australian Irlen Clinic Director's Conference. University of Newcastle, Sydney, Australia: September 27-28, 1997.

Robinson, G. L., & Foreman, P. J. (1999). Scotopic sensitivity/Irlen Syndrome and the use of colored filters: A long-term placebo controlled and masked study of reading achievement and perception of ability. *Perceptual and Motor Skills, 89,* 83-113.

Robinson, G. L., Sparkes, D. L., Roberts, T. K., & Dunstan, H. (7-11 July, 2004). *Biochemical anomalies in people with Irlen Syndrome.* University of Newcastle, NSW, Australia: Eighth International Irlen Conference, Brugge, Belgium.

Rollins, J. A. (2004). Imaging study shows differences in brain functioning in children with ADHD. *Pediatric Nursing, 30,* 165-166.

Roueche, J. E., & Roueche, S. D. (1999). *High stakes, high performance: Making remedial education work.* Washington, D. C.: Community College Press.

Rueda, M. R., Rothbart, M. K., McCandliss, B. D., Saccomanno, L., & Posner, M. I. (2005). Training, maturation, and genetic influences on the development of executive attention. *National Academy of Sciences, 102,* 14931-14936.

Salopek, J. J. (1998). Train your brain. *Training & Development, 52,* 26-34.

Samuelsson, S., & Lundberg, I. (2003). The impact of environmental factors on components of reading and dyslexia. *Annals of Dyslexia, 53,* 201-210.

Samuelsson, S., Lundberg, I., & Herkner, B. (2004). ADHD and reading disability in male adults: Is there a connection? *Journal of Learning Disabilities, 37,* 155-169.

Sands, S., & Buchholz, E. S. (1997). The underutilization of computers to assist in the remediation of dyslexia. *International Journal of Instructional Media, 24,* 153-176.

Sapolsky, R. (2000). Score one for nature—or is it nurture? *USA Today,* June 21, 17A.

Sapolsky, R. M. (2004, December). Stressed-out memories: A little stress sharpens memory, but after prolonged stress, the mental picture isn't pretty. *Scientific American Mind,* 28-33.

Schneider, M. F. (2001). (2nd Ed.). *Word Power.* New York: Simon & Schuster.

Schumacher, J., Anthoni, H., Dahdouh, F., Konig, I. R., et al. (2006). Strong genetic evidence of DCDC2 as a susceptibility gene for dyslexia. *American Journal of Human Genetics, 78,* 52-62.

Schwartz, D. (May, 2007). 'Exceptional' research: APF's 2007 Rosen grantee will explore the seldom-studied phenomenon of twice exceptionality. *Monitor on Psychology, 20*, 94.

Science News. (May 8, 2004). Words in the brain: Reading program spurs neural rewrite in kids, *165*, 291.

Sears, B. (2005). *The anti-inflammation zone: Reversing the silent epidemic that's destroying our health*. New York: HarperCollins.

Sears, B. (2002). *The omega Rx zone: The miracle of the new high-dose fish oil*. New York: Regan Books.

Shaywitz, S., M.D. (2003). *Overcoming dyslexia: A new and complete science-based program for reading problems at any level*. New York: Alfred A. Knopf.

Shaywitz, S. E., Mody, M., & Shaywitz, B. A. (2006). Neural mechanisms in dyslexia. *Current Directions in Psychological Science, 15*, 278-281.

Simonton, D. K. (2000). Creativity: Cognitive, personal, developmental, and social aspects. *American Psychologist, 55*, 151-158.

Singer, E. (2005). The strategies adopted by Dutch children with dyslexia to maintain their self-esteem when teased at school. *Journal of Learning Disabilities, 38*, 411-423.

Smith, E. E., & Jonides, J. (1999). Storage and executive processes in the frontal lobes. *Science, 283*, 1657-1661.

Solan, H. A., Shelley-Tremblay, J., Ficarra, A., Silverman, M., & Larson, S. (2003). Effect of attention therapy on reading comprehension. *Journal of Learning Disabilities, 36*, 556-565.

Spafford, C. A., & Grosser, G. S. (2005). (2nd Edition). *Dyslexia and reading difficulties: Research and resource guide for working with all struggling readers*. Boston: Pearson Education.

Spielberger, C. D., & Associates. (1977). *Test attitude inventory.* Palo Alto, CA: Consulting Psychologists Press, Inc.

Sprenger-Charolles, L., Cole, P., Lacert, P., & Serniclaes, W. (2000). On subtypes of developmental dyslexia: Evidence from processing time and accuracy scores. *Canadian Journal of Experimental Psychology, 54,* 87-104.

Stahl, S. A. (Fall, 1999). Different strokes for different folks? A critique of learning styles. *American Educator, 23,* 27-31.

Sternberg, R. J. (Spring, 1999). Ability and expertise: It's time to replace the current model of intelligence. *American Educator, 23,* 11-13, 50-51.

Sternberg, R. J. (1995). For whom the bell curve tolls: A review of the bell curve. *Psychological Science, 6,* 257-261.

Sternberg, R. J. (1996). Myths, countermyths, and truths about intelligence. *Educational Researcher, 25,* 11-16.

Sternberg, R. J. (2001). *Successful intelligence: How practical and creative intelligence determine success in life.* New York: Simon & Schuster.

Sternberg, R. J., & Grigorenko, E. L. (1999). *Our labeled children: What every parent and teacher needs to know about learning disabilities.* Cambridge, MA: Perseus Publishing.

Stevens, L. J. (2000). *12 effective ways to help your ADD / ADHD child.* New York: Avery.

Stevens, L. J., Zentall, S. S., Deck, J. L., Abate, M. L. et al. (1995). Essential fatty acid metabolism in boys with attention-deficit hyperactivity disorder. *The American Journal of Clinical Nutrition, 62,* 761-772.

Stone, R. (2002). *The light barrier: A color solution to your child's light-based reading difficulties.* New York: St. Martin's Press.

Stordy, B. J., & Nicholl, M. J. (2000). *The LCP solution: The remarkable nutritional treatment for ADHD, dyslexia, & dyspraxia.* New York: Ballantine.

Swanson, H. L. (2000). Are working memory deficits in readers with learning disabilities hard to change? *Journal of Learning Disabilities, 33*, 551-566.

Tallal, P., & Benasich, A. A. (2002). Developmental language learning impairments. *Development and Psychopathology, 14*, 559-579.

Tallal, P., Miller, S. L., Bedi, G., Byma, G., et al. (1996). Language comprehension in language-learning impaired children improved with acoustically modified speech. *Science, 271*, 81-89.

Temple, E., Poldrack, R. A., Protopapas, A., Nagarajan, S., Salz, T., Tallal, P., Merzenich, M. M., & Gabrieli, J. D. E. (2000). Disruption of the neural response to rapid acoustic stimuli in dyslexia: Evidence from functional MRI. *Proceedings of the National Academy of Science, 97*, 13907-13912.

Thomson, J. M., Richardson, U., & Goswami, U. (2005). Phonological similarity neighborhoods and children's short-term memory: Typical development and dyslexia. *Memory & Cognition, 33*, 1210-1219.

Tobias, S. (1995). *Overcoming math anxiety.* New York: W. W. Norton.

Travis, J. (1996). Let the games begin: Brain-training video games and stretched speech may help language-impaired kids and dyslexics. *Science News, 149*, 104-106.

Vastag, B. (2007). Brain gain: Constant sprouting of neurons attracts scientists, drugmakers. *Science News, 171*, 376-377, 380.

Verhaeghen, J. (2004). A working memory workout: How to expand the focus of serial attention from one to four items in 10 hours or less. *Journal of Experimental Psychology: Learning, Memory, and Cognition, 30*, 1322-1337.

Weil, A., M.D. (2000). *Eating well for optimum health: The essential guide to food, diet, and nutrition.* New York: Alfred A. Knopf.

Whiting, P. R. (1993). How difficult can reading be? *Parent & Citizen, 44*, 12-18.

Whiting, P. R. (1994-1995). Visual aspects of dyslexia. *The Bulletin for Learning Disabilities, 1 & 2,* 13-35. The Australian Institute of Learning Disabilities.

Wickelgren, I. (2001). Working memory helps the mind focus. *Science, 291,* 1684-1685.

Wilkins, A., & Smith, L. (2007). How many colours are necessary to increase the reading speed of children with visual stress? A comparison of two systems. *Journal of Research in Reading, X,* 1-12.

Willingham, D. T. (Summer, 2007). Critical thinking: Why is it so hard to teach? *American Educator, 31,* 8-19.

Willingham, D. T. (Summer, 2005). Do visual, auditory, and kinesthetic learners need visual, auditory, and kinesthetic instruction? *American Educator, 29,* 31-35, 44.

Winner, E. (2000). The origins and ends of giftedness. *American Psychologist, 55,* 159-169.

Winters, C. A. (1997). Learning disabilities, crime, delinquency, and special education placement. *Adolescence, 32,* 451-463.

Wolfe, P. (2001). *Brain matters: Translating research into classroom practice.* Alexandria, VA: Association for Supervision and Curriculum Development.

Wood, J. (2001). Can software support children's vocabulary development? *Learning & Technology, 5,* 166-201.

Worldwatch Institute. (January/February, 2000). Matters of scale: Attention deficit disorder. www.worldwatch.org/pubs/mag/2000/131/mos/

Wu, K. K., Anderson, V., & Castiello, U. (2002). Neuropsychological evaluation of deficits in executive functioning for ADHD children with or without learning disabilities. *Developmental Neuropsychology, 22,* 501-531.

Zentall, S. S. (2006). *ADHD and education: Foundations, characteristics, methods, and collaboration.* Upper Saddle River, N.J.: Pearson Education.

About the author

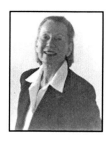

Dr. France Morrow is an interdisciplinary scholar who has taught psychology for more than two decades. In Irvine, California, Dr. Morrow taught for Pepperdine University's Graduate School of Education and Psychology and for the United States International University's Graduate Campus. Dr. Morrow has taught psychology for a Washington State college since 1994 and is an Adjunct Professor of Psychology for Washington State University. Dr. Morrow's well-received text on the psychology of gender, *Unleashing Our Unknown Selves: An Inquiry into the Future of Femininity and Masculinity* (Praeger Press, 1991) has been used in gender studies courses in several states.

For the past decade, Dr. Morrow has developed and directed successful learning programs and established a pilot study research program site under the sponsorship of the Washington State University Foundation. Dr. Morrow's central research focus is on cognition and student learning and how students' visual-perceptual and cognitive-processing difficulties can be identified and remediated through computerized skill-building exercises. This research has unfolded naturally from Dr. Morrow's previous research into brain plasticity and the ways in which the brain and central nervous system develop through social interaction.

Dr. Morrow has presented her effective learning programs at various national and international conferences including the Western Psychological Association's 1999 Conference, the University of Texas, Austin, National Institute for Staff and Organizational Development (NISOD) 1999 Conference, and many Washington State Conferences and Workshops from 1996 to the present, including her 2006 Washington State University Learning Program Workshop designed for Washington State K-12 educators.

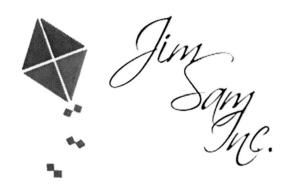

Please visit our website at
www.JimSamInc.com
to order additional copies.

JimSam Inc. Publishing
P.O. Box 3363
Riverview, FL 33568
813.748.9523

Printed in the United States
203578BV00004B/1-146/P

9 780979 076862